Interprofessional Consultation

Innovation and Imagination in Working Relationships

Derek Steinberg
MB,BS(Lond),MPhil(Lond),DPM,FRCPsych
*Consultant Psychiatrist, The Maudsley Hospital
and Bethlem Royal Hospital, London
Honorary Visiting Reader in Psychiatry and Human
Development, University of Surrey, Guildford*

Illustrations by the author

BLACKWELL SCIENTIFIC PUBLICATIONS

OXFORD LONDON EDINBURGH

BOSTON MELBOURNE

Blackwell Scientific Publications
Editorial offices:
Osney Mead, Oxford OX2 0EL
  (*Orders*: Tel. 0865 240201)
8 John Street, London WC1N 2ES
23 Ainslie Place, Edinburgh EH3 6AJ
3 Cambridge Center, Suite 208
  Cambridge, Massachusetts 02142, USA
107 Barry Street, Carlton
  Victoria 3053, Australia

First published 1989

Set by DP Photosetting, Aylesbury, Bucks
Printed and bound in Great Britain by
Mackays of Chatham PLC, Chatham, Kent

DISTRIBUTORS

USA
  Year Book Medical Publishers
  200 North LaSalle Street,
  Chicago, Illinois 60601
  (*Orders*: Tel. (312) 726-9733)

Canada
  The C.V. Mosby Company
  5240 Finch Avenue East
  Scarborough, Ontario
  (*Orders*: Tel. 416 298-1588)

Australia
  Blackwell Scientific Publications
  (Australia) Pty Ltd
  107 Barry Street
  Carlton, Victoria 3053
  (*Orders*: Tel. (03) 347-0300)

British Library
Cataloguing in Publication Data
Steinberg, Derek
  Interprofessional consultation.
  1. Professional personnel. Communication
  I. Title
  658.3'044

ISBN 0-632-02252-3

Contents

Foreword

by Denise Taylor, Formerly Principal Psychologist and Founding Organising Tutor, Advanced Course in Consultation, Tavistock Clinic, London

This practical, introductory guide to consultative work will be welcomed by health care and educational professionals. The increasingly complex problems thrown up by society are reflected in the growth of legal, organisational and ethical issues confronting a growing range of specialists and agencies and make co-operation between different kinds of professional workers both more essential and more difficult.

As Dr Steinberg points out, consultation is a joint exercise in problem clarification and problem solving which enhances the professional competence of consultees as well as helping them to learn how to consult to others. The consultant and consultee have a co-equal relationship, where each respects the other's expertise, and where a climate is created which enables each to achieve the 'courage of one's own stupidity', as Michael Balint put it – in other words, where seemingly naive questions can be asked and established professional presumptions can be temporarily put aside to allow the situation to be looked at anew. While the basic principles of consultation are straightforward and uncontroversial, it can make a 'difference that matters' in Gregory Bateson's sense of the term and the implications can be radical.

These and other important issues in consultation are discussed and illustrated by Dr Steinberg in the context of his own extensive experience and theoretical framework. This book is a welcome addition to the literature on consultation in this country for the helping professions.

Denise Taylor

Preface

The term consultation is a familiar one because so many people use it, though in many different ways. A patient consults a doctor; a doctor consults another doctor; a commercial company employs a team of consultants; a staff union leader consults the membership; an administrator consults colleagues about an aspect of the organisation.

But what does consultation mean? Like the terms psychotherapy, or counselling, it suggests different things to different people. This need not be a bad thing during the evolution of a particular method; something akin to natural selection operates, approaches and terminology are polished up and refined or become redundant, and in due course we come to know what each other is talking about when we use a particular word.

The point of this book is to describe and identify – as interprofessional consultation – a particular way of working which, I believe, deserves definition. How useful the approach happens to be is another question; but if we describe it and name it we are at least on the road to evaluating it too.

By interprofessional consultation I mean the work undertaken when one person (the consultant) helps another (the consultee) to do his or her work without taking it over; the consultee retains control of work in hand, the methods used, and responsibility for it too. This preliminary definition is perhaps unremarkable, but contains the seeds of the reasons why this sort of consultation differs from others.

Interprofessional consultation, at one level, is one way of A helping B with a specified question. It may be a problem, even a crisis, or it may be simply a matter of consulting about how best to proceed concerning a particular development.

At a more complex level, it is also about how specialists can talk usefully to each other, bringing their respective experience and skill to bear on something which may concern, say, a client, a student, a pupil or a patient, or on an organisational or academic issue.

Interprofessional consultation, by these sorts of definition, is identified as one form of collaborative work. But there are other ways of collaborating which are quite different, and this is discussed in the first chapter. And having very broadly established what is meant by consultation in *this* book, I will, for the sake of brevity, drop the qualification 'interprofessional' in most of the rest of the text.

Much of my own work is in child and adolescent psychiatry, and in teaching and training in these fields and in the creative psychotherapies, so many of the examples given in this book are drawn from these subjects. However, I hope it will seem to the reader that the basic principles of the consultative approach have a much wider application.

A further point on the use of words. Consultation is often to do with aspects of work which involve counselling, treatment, teaching and administration. For simplicity, I have used the word clinical to distinguish various forms of therapeutic and counselling work from teaching, organising and so on, even though I realise it isn't always precisely right to do so.

It can take newcomers to the theory and practice of consultation a little time to appreciate the essential *equality* in the consultative relationship. So much in the clinical, care, administrative and teaching fields is concerned with A telling B what to do, albeit disguised in various ways, that the extent to which consultative work is a process of shared exploration of the matter in hand may not be apparent at first sight. 'To consult' is the word for what both consultant and consultee do, and both require skill to undertake it.

Derek Steinberg
The Maudsley Hospital, London, and
Bethlem Royal Hospital, Beckenham, Kent.

Acknowledgements

I would like to acknowledge the teaching of Denise Taylor, Dorothy Heard, Harold Bridger and the late Irene Caspari of the Tavistock Clinic and Institute's training programme in consultation and community mental health; the seminars on consultation and attachment theory which developed out of this course, and were led by Dorothy Heard and John Bowlby; work and discussion with Christopher Dare, Bill Yule, Lynette Hughes and Carol Sheldrick at the Maudsley Hospital and Institute of Psychiatry and with Rosemary Ryle and Peter Wilson from the associated Camberwell Clinic and the London Youth Advisory Centre respectively; John Foskett, Chaplain to the Maudsley and Bethlem Royal Hospitals, convenor of the Hospitals' Training Group on staff working relationships and leader of the staff group in my own unit; Michael Woods and his colleagues at Adelaide House Children's Home in North Kensington; further afield, the staff at the Ministry of Community Development, Republic of Singapore, and in particular Major Tan Keng Hiang, Mrs Janet Yee, Miss M. Menon and Miss Ang Bee Lian; and Dr Wong Sze Tai, Director of the Child Psychiatric Service in Singapore; all for their generous hospitality as well as for the many opportunities for discussion and learning; similarly, thanks to Dr Joaquin Fuentes Biggi and staff of the Ministry of Health of the Basque Government, San Sebastian, Spain; Professor P. Sakellaropoulos and colleagues at the University of Thrace and in the community psychiatric service based in Alexandroupolis, Greece; Dr Ritsa Papatheophilou of the Adolescent Psychiatric Service at Athens General Hospital;

Katerina Robertson and Giorgos Polos of the Arts and Therapy Centre, Athens; Dr Sue Jennings of the Institute for Arts and Therapy, London; Joanna Beazley Richards; and Jafar Kareem and Dr Sarangshou Acharyya of NAFSIYAT, the Inter-Cultural Therapy Centre, London. The experience of working with them and their organisations is behind many of the ideas and the anecdotes in this book, and to all of them I owe my thanks.

D.S.

A note on confidentiality

Confidentiality is more of a problem in consultation than it is in clinical work. It is always possible to disguise the identity of a patient, but it is far more difficult to hide the identity of an institution. For this reason, the examples given in the text are fictitious, although authentic in principle, except in some cases where it is clear from the nature of the example that confidentiality would be unnecessary.

For Gill, Anna and Kate

Chapter 1

Introduction: What is Consultation?

Address, advise, articulate, assess, attend to, bargain, blather, brief, chat to, communicate, converse, confer, convene, consult, chew the rag, collaborate, command, commend, contribute, consider, counsel, debate, declaim, diagnose, discuss, dictate, direct, discourse, empathise, encourage, entreat, examine, exhort, explain, exchange, gossip, guide, handle, harangue, hearken, heed, hint, hold forth, inform, influence, instruct, interrogate, interview, lecture, lend an ear, liaise, listen, manage, meet, narrate, natter, negotiate, orate, order, oversee, persuade, press, propose, pursue, question, rant, reappraise, reconsider, request, require, review, say, see, share, speak, submit, support, suggest, supervise, talk, teach, treat, utter, verbalise, witter.

Consultation: introduction

A great deal of talking goes on in the therapeutic and 'helping' professions. Consultation is the sort of talk undertaken when one person (the consultant) helps another (the consultee – or a group of consultees) to work effectively, but without taking that work over in any way. To use a piece of jargon which I don't like, but which I think will help convey the nature of consultative work, the purpose of the consultant is to *facilitate* the work of the consultees. To use another, the consultant acts as *enabler*.

The problem of finding the right word is itself interesting. As I hope what follows will show, there is nothing quite like consultation, although many things are similar. Hence consultation often gets muddled with such activities as supervision, psychotherapy, liaison work and so on. In this chapter I will try to show the differences between consultation and other work, and then demonstrate, I hope, why the distinction is worth making.

One of the problems is that the term consultant is already used for all sorts of other roles; and the fact is that the proponents of consultation as defined here have hijacked this general term for our own specialised purposes. This usurping of a word is one of the few imperious acts in what is otherwise, and by definition, an essentially friendly and user-orientated enterprise. Suggestions for a better term would be welcome. Meanwhile, those who want to learn about consultation should appreciate that, for example, consultants in the National Health Service often aren't consultants in the sense used here, while the work of a management consultant can again be different, for example to assess a situation and then provide advice or even quite specific recommendations. All this is like consultation, and related to it, but lacks the core characteristics of consultative work as described here.

The consultative perspective

The key difference between consultation, in the sense used here, and other forms of interprofessional talk, is that the perspective taken is primarily that of the other person.

In much of what goes on in the therapeutic, counselling, diagnostic, remedial, 'helping' and administrative professions, there is a more or less overt effort to persuade the other person to see or do things the way the first person wants. Thus the psychotherapist has a number of personal assumptions about what is reasonable, right or normal, and the teacher and the manager have preconceptions about the right or best way for the other person to proceed. Often this is as it should be; if I need a technical job done properly, whether it is a roof repair or an appendicectomy, a fire extinguished or a carpet laid, I would like to leave it to the experts. The same applies to many aspects of medical care, not excluding some aspects of psychiatry and some forms of psychotherapy.

Consultation is different. Consultative work is about working with *other people's* perspectives, assumptions and expertise. To do this requires something of an act of faith in the consultee (up to a point: see later) and a measure of self-discipline too. It is common among those training in consultative work only partly to accept this crucial point, and doctors and psychodynamic psychotherapists have particular trouble here. The doctor, as consultant, sets out with every intention to leave responsibility for the task in hand with the consultee, but at the first appearance of difficulty or anxiety there is a tendency for the doctor to take on some of the responsibility, a development in which the consultee may well collude. The psychotherapist, working as a consultant, tries to help the consultee frame and clarify matters in his own way, but finds himself drawn towards psychodynamic notions of what is going on, in terms of private beliefs about the consultee's personality, feelings, motivations and defence mechanisms.

We will return to these and other difficulties in this work after considering some basic definitions and guidelines.

Consultation: towards a definition

What distinguishes consultation from other types of joint work are some key characteristics (Caplan, 1970; Steinberg and Yule 1985) which will be listed briefly here, and discussed and elaborated later.

(1) The consultant works through the consultee, rather than directly with the problem or question in hand.
(2) It is the consultee's perceptions, understanding, skills and methods which are primarily used to deal with the matter in hand, not those of the consultant. Much of this involves the consultee widening his or her perspectives and reframing ideas and attitudes.
(3) The consultee remains responsible for the work being discussed; the consultant does not take over or share this responsibility.
(4) The consultee remains autonomous. He or she decides how, if at all, to use what emerges from the consultation.
(5) It is assumed that the consultee is a fully competent worker within the limits of his or her status and role, and that the latter is appropriate to the matter being discussed.

(6) Professional training and development are regarded as integral to consultative work. Acceptance by consultant and consultee of the above guidelines means that the consultee will learn something new from the exercise, and will therefore be in a better position to manage future problems.
(7) Consultation should be a pragmatic, helpful exercise. In the interests of this it is sometimes sensible, even necessary, to bend or break the above rules, provided that their general spirit is understood and followed.

A guide to the following chapters

All the special characteristics as well as the variety of consultative work follow from these few basic rules, and each needs some discussion and qualification. This is the subject matter of Chapter 2, in which the processes and content of consultation are described, leading to the elaboration in Chapter 3 of a basic model to use in consultative work.

In Chapters 4 to 6 examples of these various types of consultation are discussed, with examples drawn from different settings. The closing chapters are concerned with some wider aspects of consultative approaches, including ethical issues, evaluation and some thoughts on the role of a consultative style in holistic medical practice.

Consultation in relation to other activities

Consultation, it is being argued, is *different*. Different from what, and how? Figure 1.1 illustrates some other talking activities which overlap with consultation, those which are quite different, and those which so to speak touch upon it.

(1) Supervision

The difference between consultation and supervision commonly causes confusion, not least because the term supervision is used in two quite different ways.

Supervision in a hierarchical sense, where the supervisor is senior to the people being supervised, more experienced in the

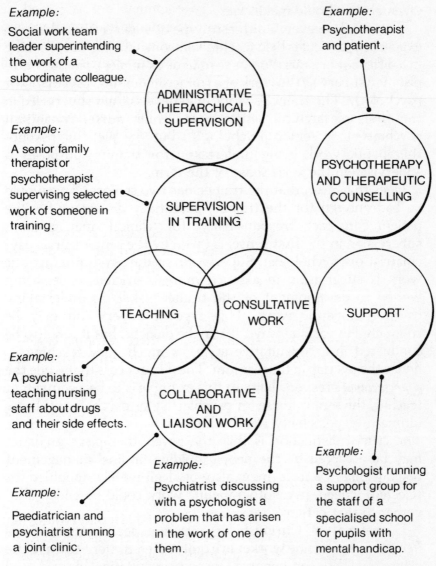

Example:

Social work team leader superintending the work of a subordinate colleague.

Example:

A senior family therapist or psychotherapist supervising selected work of someone in training.

Example:

A psychiatrist teaching nursing staff about drugs and their side effects.

Example:

Paediatrician and psychiatrist running a joint clinic.

Example:

Psychiatrist discussing with a psychologist a problem that has arisen in the work of one of them.

Example:

Psychotherapist and patient.

Example:

Psychologist running a support group for the staff of a specialised school for pupils with mental handicap.

ADMINISTRATIVE (HIERARCHICAL) SUPERVISION

SUPERVISION IN TRAINING

PSYCHOTHERAPY AND THERAPEUTIC COUNSELLING

TEACHING

CONSULTATIVE WORK

'SUPPORT'

COLLABORATIVE AND LIAISON WORK

Figure 1.1 Consultation in relation to other types of professional work.

work being done, and who takes some responsibility for their performance, ought to be clearly distinct from consultation. However, there has been a long quasi-democratic period in many areas of health and care work, with some staff uncomfortable about having a boss or being one, and the authority of the supervisor has sometimes been challenged or blurred. Hierarchical supervision, however, whether autocratic, well-balanced or fudged, is not the same as consultation, as the basic guidelines given above should make clear.

There is, however, a different type of supervision, where an expert in a particular field teaches someone who may be working in a different organisation or team. For example, a psychotherapist may supervise the work of a trainee in nursing, psychiatry or psychology. The trainee's work in general is then supervised in the first, hierarchical sense by a senior nurse, consultant psychiatrist or senior psychologist; but the piece of psychotherapeutic work being undertaken for training purposes is supervised in the *second* sense of the term.

Does this mean that the trainee has two seniors? This would be bad enough for the trainee, potentially disastrous for the patient. In fact, responsibility for clinical management, supervision in the first sense, is taken by the senior nurse, psychiatrist or psychologist. Supervision of the psychotherapeutic work is supervision in a much more restricted sense, being limited to development of the trainee's skills in undertaking psychotherapeutic work. This type of supervision may be conducted in various ways: it may be didactic, but it can also be conducted in a consultative style, as much good teaching is, hence the overlap in the diagram. The difference is that while the *psychotherapist's* responsibility in this example is to be a competent teacher, the senior nurse (or psychiatrist, or psychologist) bears ultimate responsibility for the junior's work with the patient. The crucial distinction is this: the psychotherapist's guidance may be accepted by the people holding 'in-line' management responsibility; but it may also be legitimately modified or rejected; indeed, psychotherapeutic work could be ended altogether in that patient's case.

Does it matter? Curiously, organisations seeking consultative help from an outside worker are quite often content to leave the distinction between supervision and consultation blurred, and the consultant who tries to clarify this may feel that he or she is splitting hairs. But the difference is very important, as becomes clear if you ask the simple question: who is responsible if something goes wrong? The supervisor in the hierarchy is responsible, not the consultant, whose responsibility is limited to providing competent and ethically sound consultative help. (What sometimes happens when this key issue is explored in some organisations is the revelation that no-one is clearly in charge; this is itself a potentially helpful discovery and one that

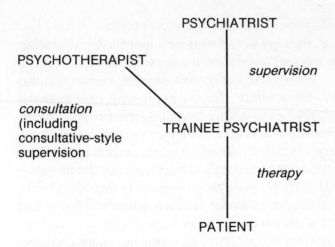

Figure 1.2 Supervision in relation to consultation: an example of a psychotherapist providing consultation to a trainee psychiatrist. (N.B. if the psychotherapist were providing formal, systematic psychotherapy supervision it would be no less necessary to clarify the respective positions of psychiatrist, psychotherapist and trainee along the above lines.)

incidentally illustrates the usefulness of the consultative approach.)

From a wider perspective, clarity about the respective roles of senior manager as supervisor and consultant as teacher enables the specialised (e.g. psychological) skills of the latter to be made available to an organisation, widening the scope of its thinking, teaching and practice, but without complicating the lines of management and authority.

(2) Psychotherapy

On the face of it psychotherapy ought not to become confused with consultative work; psychotherapy is about treating people's personal problems and disorders, consultation is about people's work. In practice confusion is common, and the person taking a consultative group may be surprised to overhear the session described as a 'therapy group', sometimes months after he thought the matter had been clarified.

There are three reasons for this common misunderstanding:

First, many workers in the psychiatric, psychological and social work fields arrange to receive psychotherapy to help with their personal feelings and relationships, in order, among other things, to cope with their demanding work or to do it better. This notion of being 'in therapy' for the sake of their work is laudable, but it is often unclear whether it is being undertaken for personal reasons (treatment) or professional reasons ('training therapy'). Many argue that the distinction is unimportant, regarding therapy as something that is good for everyone's normal development, which I consider a contradiction in terms. Whatever the arguments, however, it commonly happens that when a staff member or group sees a consultant for the purposes of exploring work difficulties, which necessarily includes discussion of feelings, attitudes and relationships, some will think they are undergoing a therapeutic exercise.

Second, the notion of 'support' in work becomes confused with consultation and hence again with psychotherapy. The argument, implied more than explicit, commonly goes something like this: people are weak (shades of High Priesthood) and have vulnerabilities which the stresses and strains of work in the psychosocial fields shows up, and therefore 'support groups' are needed to help them struggle through the working week.

In my view, the argument should really run as follows: the demands made on staff by clientele, by the community and often by the organisation are commonly excessive and quite unreasonable, and a constant theme of professional work should be to do with the question: What is being asked of me? What is the most appropriate way of responding? How should I manage my time and energy to respond helpfully, and with what resources? These sorts of questions have been dealt with realistically by soldiers, sailors, engineers, manufacturers, farmers and others for many years, but in general the psychosocial, 'helping' professions tend not to ask such questions of themselves and their colleagues, except in 'therapy', and not surprisingly soon feel in need of 'support'.

Of course it is friendly to be supportive, whatever the task in hand, and staff may well find consultation supportive in a general way, just as a good teaching programme, proper meal breaks and a stimulating and friendly atmosphere are all sustaining in their different ways. But a consultative session is not primarily a 'support group', although, if you check, you will not infrequently find that it is thought to be one. The difference is this: a 'support group' takes the task and the work for granted, and seeks to help people to cope emotionally with it. A consultative group raises questions about the task and the way it is being handled. If it is *also* supportive that is fine, and a useful side effect.

The third reason is that the processes involved in group and individual consultation can be very similar to some forms of psychotherapy, although by no means all. Thus there are some similarities with Rogerian-type psychotherapy or counselling (Rogers, 1951) precisely because it emphasises the therapist helping the client find his own solutions in his own way; on the other hand, many schools of psychotherapy adhere to their own quite complex models of understanding, no more accessible to the client than biochemistry. Thus dynamic psychotherapy, with its concern with unconscious motivation, is quite different from consultation. Caplan (1970) pointed out the difficulties psycho-analytically trained psychotherapists can have with consultative work, with their preoccupation with unconscious motivation, defensive manoeuvres and a tendency to ask 'why?' something is happening, when the appropriate questions in consultative work are about *what* is happening.

In clearing space for itself, so to speak, consultation has to contend with real practical and conceptual problems to do with distinguishing from each other (a) the treatment of disorder, (b) the enhancement of personal development, and (c) the essentially educational task of helping with professional development. It is one of the interesting characteristics of the theory and practice of consultation that it does seek clarity about questions like these, which have long been somewhat hedged for under-standable historical and professional reasons.

It would be convenient if consultation could be clearly distinguished from counselling, but there is a problem in making a completely clear distinction between consultation and that type of counselling which acknowledges the autonomy and potential for effective self-management of the other person. This is a conceptual problem brought about by real cultural and social changes in the relationships between specialist workers and those who use their help, so that the user of specialist services is increasingly seen as someone seeking education rather than needing rescue. Accordingly, a more realistic distinction between psychotherapy, counselling and consultation may require draw-ing the dividing line through counselling itself, and distinguish-ing between that which follows the somewhat paternalistic or maternalistic therapeutic tradition, and that which operates more as a peer-peer exercise. Both have their place, but the latter is closer to consultation, even though the focus is on a personal rather than a work issue.

This discussion is taken further in relation to developments in holistic medicine and health care in Chapter 8.

(3) Teaching

Teaching is easier to relate to consultative work, because consultation is generally conducted as an exercise from which everyone involved learns, using everyday work experiences and issues great or small as teaching material. Thus consultation may be set up in the form of a regular, in-service training programme in which staff bring to the session matters arising from their work and from which they can learn; or, conversely, *ad hoc* or emergency consultative meetings held specifically to deal with a crisis or problem can be handled in such a way that everyone involved learns something for next time from the experience.

Consultation, particularly when arranged for an organisation or team on a regular basis, is therefore likely to contribute to staff training. Conversely, one method of teaching is to ask the student to think through the nature of the question and the possible solutions, and then to select from the possible alternatives. This non-didactic method of teaching comes very close to the consultative approach.

(4) Collaborative and liaison work

Collaborative and liaison work similarly overlap with consultative work, in that consultation is one way of carrying out either. Accounts of collaborative and liaison work in psychiatry may be found in Gelder *et al.* (1985) and Gomez (1986) and in paediatrics and child psychiatry in Mrazek (1985).

Gelder *et al.* (1985) distinguish between consultation work, when the psychiatrist is available to give an opinion on patients referred to him, and liaison work, where the psychiatrist becomes part of the medical or surgical team, taking part in ward rounds and clinical meetings and offering advice on any patient to whose care he feels able to contribute. Consultation in these definitions clearly means clinical consultation, with assessment of the patient being part of the service offered. Mrazek (1985) gives a helpful account of a number of ways in which psychiatrists and paediatricians may consult together, but without delineating interprofessional consultation as defined in this chapter.

Clearly there is much potential for misunderstanding in the field, and perhaps the best single piece of advice for the aspiring consultant (or liaison worker) is always to make sure that he knows precisely what those seeking his help want him to do, and that he is able and willing to respond.

Example: A senior anaesthetic registrar in an intensive care unit asks her psychiatric counterpart to provide consultation to the unit, because of the high levels of stress among the unit's staff and the large number of psychiatric problems in the patients under their care. The willing SR checks with his own senior and with the consultant physician in charge of the unit, and gets encouragement to proceed from each.

The psychiatric SR considers that the first meeting was a good start. Problems of handling the feelings of patients and their relatives, dealing with staff feelings in the face of anxiety and death, problems of communication and authority, responsibility and failure and the roles of the many different specialists involved in each patient's care are discussed.

The senior nurse appears, and asks to see the SR. She doesn't want her staff psychoanalysed, thank you very much; she once worked on a psychiatric unit and has seen all the time wasted on groups, and all the damage done.

The next day, a Friday, the psychiatric SR's senior is discomfited to learn that three 'overdoses' in the Intensive Care Unit have been placed under his care, by virtue of his senior registrar's role there, and the physician in charge would like them discharged or transferred to a psychiatric ward before the weekend, 'to make room for emergencies'.

Muddles and misunderstandings of this type are by no means uncommon. Indeed, as will be explained later, the first step in consultative work is to clarify what is wanted by whom and with what authority.

Suggested terminology

Collaborative work

This means no more nor less than working together. It may refer to consultative work or any form of liaison work, and need have no more specific, technical meaning.

Liaison work

This refers to regular collaboration between workers or teams whose methods, objectives and focus of work is ordinarily different. Hence the advantage gained is of bringing in an additional perspective, for example if a psychiatrist joins in a diabetic clinic or a paediatrician's ward round, or a neurologist works with a psychiatrist who sees a large number of patients with epilepsy. It may involve clinical consultation or interprofessional consultation, or both.

The value of consultation

What is there about consultation's potential, to justify such careful delineation from other activities?

(1) It can help a proportion (perhaps a large one) of patients or clients who might otherwise be re-referred to specialists to stay with their original 'front-line' worker instead.

(2) Conversely, it should assist the process by which patients or clients are referred to more specialised help only when this is really necessary, and clarify the reasons for doing so.

(3) A shared reappraisal of the extent to which the first, 'front-line' or referring practitioner has the expertise to manage his client's problem after all is appropriate for very large numbers of the problems referred to psychiatrists and psychologists. Often this would not be appropriate for, say, many medical or surgical problems.

For example, meningitis or acute appendicitis are each diagnosed by specific symptoms and signs, and meningitis can be confirmed by specialised tests. Both require special facilities for their management. The same is true for some serious psychiatric conditions, such as acute psychotic illness.

In the case of emotional and behavioural problems it is by no means clear or universally agreed what the best response should be, nor who is best qualified to provide it. For example 'behaviour problems' in a school pupil may hypothetically be helped by behaviour therapy, by individual counselling or psychotherapy, by social casework with the parents, or by family therapy. Much of this broadly psychosocial and educational approach is quite often within the broad scope of the person considering making a referral. Indeed, they may well have tried one or other approach, and for some reason abandoned it, assumed it will not be sufficiently helpful, or lost confidence in what they were doing.

Such problems constitute some 90 per cent of those that are referred to child and adolescent psychiatrists. The situation is comparable in psychiatry generally. It is not possible, at least not yet, to say that one person should go to a psychotherapist, another to a psychologist, another to a psychiatrist, with the same confidence with which, say, a general practitioner would refer the patient with appendicitis to a surgeon and the child with meningitis to a hospital physician. There is therefore good reason for suggesting that when an individual's behaviour or feelings cause concern it is worth exploring consultatively with the front-line worker what he or she has tried and whether there is a case for pressing on, perhaps in the same way or perhaps in a modified way, with help and encouragement from the consultant; or (as decided within the consultation) going to someone else, because this still remains an option.

(4) It follows from this that consultation has a function in advancing professional education and development. A residential care team, for example, who thought they could not manage a child with his problems, are helped to work out strategies for doing so. This helps them as a team and as individuals to meet future similar problems better. This would not be achieved by the child simply attending sessions in a clinic, still less if he were transferred elsewhere.

(5) The questions explored in consultation are necessarily basic ones. It is not automatically taken for granted, for example that 'depression' or even 'overdosing' have the status of appendicitis or meningitis, and necessarily indicate the need for transfer to more specialised care. The consultee and consultant can examine together such questions as what is needed by that person in the present situation, who potentially could provide it, and what

facilities they would need. For example, it may be that a patient would need admission to hospital not because they were all that ill, but because a young people's home or hostel lacked the staffing, supervision and confidence to care for the individual concerned. It may be that nothing could be done about that in the short term, but for future reference this sort of observation is worth making.

Summary and concluding note

Consultation between professional workers is quite different from clinical consultation, where the specialist takes over the care of a referred 'case'. In consultation the consultant helps the consultee explore for himself what he may still be able to do for his patient, client or pupil, so that referral to another person may prove to be unnecessary; or, if it is, the reasons should then be more clear and precise, to everyone's advantage.

Clarification of how the 'front line' professional can manage after all is likely to show or remind him or her of personal resources he or she wasn't using to the full, or indicate new ways of understanding the problem or new management strategies. In this sense consultation enhances professional education and development. It may equally demonstrate what is missing in an institution or organisation, or what is not being used: there may be inadequate training, staffing or supervision, for example. Good consultation is likely to be educational in more ways than one, as well as problem-solving and supportive. Nonetheless, it is to be distinguished from related activities, with which it is sometimes confused, such as teaching, supervision or psychotherapy.

Consultation is therefore educational. It also provides in a unique way a joint method of enquiry into the fundamental nature of problems and ways of responding to them. In so far as it is conducted effectively, it enables people in difficulties to stay with their front-line helpers (who become more skilled) rather than become transferred to the care of new and more specialised people, and thereby transformed into patients. When individuals do need specialised technical expertise, however, the consultative process, far from hindering the referral process, helps enable it to be appropriate. This is particularly important in the psychosocial field, where referral and re-referral is commonly arbitrary and unhelpful, so that it may take a great deal of time and effort for the most suitable help to be delivered to the right place. The time spent in consultation – perhaps a few minutes, perhaps an hour – is likely to be considerably less than the time and resources wasted by the wrong help being delivered at the wrong time and in the wrong place.

Here is the essential difference: in the traditional model, A has a more or less vague idea of B's problems, and of C's facilities and skills, and accordingly arranges for B to be seen by C.

In the consultative model, A talks to C to see what each can do to help. In the process of joint exploration of the problem A and C discover more about the nature of the problem and about what each other have to offer B.

Chapter 2

The Consultative Process: Basic Principles

Consultation: the basic principles of aim, form and approach

Consultative work is simple in its basic principles, complex in its forms and implications. In this chapter the basic points will be examined from the following perspectives:

(1) When is consultation useful?
(2) Who may be involved in consultation? What forms may it take?
(3) What areas of work are there to be covered in consultation?

(1) When is consultation useful?

The simple answer is: when the main need is not so much for the consultant's technical knowledge or skill, but about how best to apply that of the consultee. In all fields we have countless methods and variations of methods at our disposal: the prescription of a drug, the use of one or other psychotherapy, the adoption of a style of teaching, the introduction of a particular form of administration. What we do not have is much in the way of certainty about which is best; and even when there seems to be some scientific or quasi-scientific evidence that a particular approach is 'best', there are still questions of personal opinion, personal choice, practicalities, economics and ethics to be considered.

To take one example: I believe it is as certain as anything can be that the surest way to help someone with a schizophrenic illness is by using one of the phenothiazine drugs. I would not want to treat a patient I believed to have an active schizophrenic illness if for some reason the patient and relatives withheld consent for medication; because I would not know how else to treat him.

But there is another side to the issue. Although there are now agreed international criteria for the illness, that doesn't mean the diagnosis – confirming the definite presence or definite absence of the condition – can always be made; nor is it invariably clear, in all circumstances, when the risks of the side-effects of the drugs used are justified by the risks of not prescribing medication. People and circumstances and indeed the course of psychiatric disorders vary too much for there to be hard and fast rules about that. Suppose a specialised community were set up to care for people with schizophrenic and schizophrenic-like illnesses (the distinction is not always so easily made) and they got by, perhaps by having large numbers of dedicated staff, a conscientiously supervised and caring community, and the patients and their families happened not to be anxious for swift symptom-suppression and a return to the outside world?

The point I am making is that even in one of the somewhat more certain areas of psychiatry there is not only room for doubts, questions and negotiation, but a need for it. In other areas of psychiatry and health care generally things are even more open for shared evaluation of the risks, the options and the benefits of different courses of action.

Consider the following questions:

(1) The head teacher of a therapeutic school for disturbed children: 'Would it be a good idea to introduce behaviour modification principles to the school?'
(2) The senior staff of a children's home: 'We're experiencing a high rate of disturbance among the children and a lot of strain among the staff. What should we do?'
(3) The senior management of a psychiatric unit: 'We don't think we're doing enough for our patients. Is there more that we could do?'
(4) The staff of a home for elderly handicapped people: 'We want to add dramatherapy to what we do here. Can you help us do it?'
(5) The visiting psychiatrist to a therapeutic hostel: 'We've had to call the police in to one of our residents; he keeps getting

drunk and aggressive; he can't look after himself at the moment; some of the staff are going to walk out if he stays; shouldn't he be in hospital?'

The first answer to these questions, and countless questions like them, comes down to: it depends on what you want, what you've got, and what the alternatives are. Such things are by no means immediately clear.

Consultation is appropriate when those involved agree that discussion, perhaps accompanied by negotiation and various styles of joint exploration (of which more later) is the best way of sorting out how to proceed with a particular question or problem. It requires consent, and indeed informed consent, because it is important that people know what they are entering into when they accept consultative help. It is a joint exercise in problem-clarifying and problem-resolving. It may lead to problem-sharing, but on a planned basis (A contributing this and B contributing that) rather than on an arbitrary basis.

In Chapter 1 it was pointed out that the special usefulness of consultation was as an exercise that helped the clientele stay with the original workers, who learned something in the process. There is a fundamental circularity to the consultative approach (Figure 2.1) which gives it a dual-function and dual value: the primary aim can be to deal with a problem or resolve a crisis, with the consultees advancing their skills and experience in the process. Conversely, the primary aim can be educational, but with consultation about a real and current issue as the exercise in which learning takes place.

The crisis as a focus of consultation needs some explanation. Crisis means a decisive moment or turning point (Greek – *krisis*) and is by no means necessarily a sudden emergency or a bad thing. A critical period can be a time of growth as well as difficulty. One therefore refers to 'crises, problems or issues' to span the very different matters with which consultative work can usefully deal. Further, whether the point in question is a crisis or not will often depend on one's point of view. One man's plan may be someone's opportunity, someone else's minor problem and another person's crisis. To take an example, a decision to introduce an in-service training programme for (say) teachers, residential social workers or nursing staff on an in-patient unit can be tremendously destabilising in terms of work and status expectations, personal timetables and organisational

Primarily for dealing with
crises, problems or other
issues – with learning and
professional development as
an expected secondary effect.

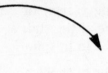

CONSULTATION

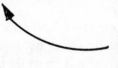

Primarily for educational and
training purposes – using
crises, problems or other
issues as material from which
to learn.

Figure 2.1 Consultation: interaction between problem-solving and educational functions.

programmes, however beneficial the overall aim may be.

With such things in mind, here are some examples of consultative work, in no particular order of importance or frequency.

- The staff of a psychiatric unit wish to change their approach from in-patient treatment to developing into a community-oriented, family therapeutic service, and seek the help of an outside consultant to help them plan and carry out this change.
- A general practice wants to improve its counselling work with patients, and asks for someone to work with the practice team for a time on a consultative basis to help develop their skills.
- A psychiatric team finds a most complex situation referred to them. There is a woman who is chronically depressed and has epilepsy, and her husband is recurrently drunk and violent. The children's ages range from 6 months to 22 years, the older children living with nearby in-laws who often have violent arguments with the parents. Several of the children are involved with school psychological and welfare services. The parents are already involved with family welfare and social services offices and also with the psychotherapist on the psychiatric team of a teaching hospital in the same district. One of the teenage daughters is depressed and behaving badly and is referred to an adolescent psychiatric unit. It is agreed, however, that instead of simply giving her an appointment a consultative meeting with the other professionals involved would be the best first step, and this is arranged urgently.

- A paediatrician would like to work in liaison with a child psychiatrist but isn't sure what sort of mutual roles and arrangements would be best. She consults the child psychiatrist about what he has to offer and what she sees as her patients' and her team's needs.
- A medical team dealing with severely and terminally ill patients seeks consultation sessions with a psychologist about the feelings that are regularly generated in their work, and which they believe they could be handling more effectively.
- A child psychiatric team has frequent referrals of young people from local children's homes. The team decides to offer a consultative service to the children's homes' staff, as well as ordinary clinical appointments.
- A social worker phones a community nurse to ask her to deal urgently with an acute problem he feels he cannot handle. The nurse, in talking through with the social worker the nature of the problem and the alternative ways of dealing with it, enables him to manage after all.
- A hospital general manager would like to see organisational skills developed among his staff. He considers a course involving lectures and seminars, but instead decides upon a weekend course in which personnel bring for consultation some examples of current administrative problems.
- A general psychiatrist is the third clinician in line trying to treat a patient with anorexia nervosa who is extremely ambivalent about receiving help, and this is generating a great deal of anxiety and uncertainty among the clinical workers as well as her relatives. On a Friday afternoon she is discovered to have been expertly disguising her weight loss, and is in a much worse physical state than the clinical team had supposed. Her relatives are furious and alarmed, and the team refer her for immediate transfer to a fourth hospital. The team at the latter, however, resist an immediate transfer on the grounds that there is every reason to believe that they risk being the fourth team likely to fail, and instead suggest consultation with the third before proceeding with any clinical plans.
- A specialised therapy centre (e.g. a dramatherapy teaching unit, or a child abuse clinic) invites a psychiatrist to help with its teaching programme. The centre and its students are likely to be more expert than the psychiatrist in their own subject;

the psychiatrist, as consultant, brings to the sessions consultative skills plus a shared understanding with the students of the context (e.g. mental health, psychodynamic psychology, child development) in which their work and training operates.

- A psychiatric team seeks the consultative help of a psychotherapist to improve the training of its staff in the psychodynamics of individual work. The therapist leads a weekly consultative seminar to which staff bring examples of their work as foci for discussion and learning. The session is not supervisory; indeed, both supervisor and supervised attend the meeting and take away from it ideas for their respective work, so that both the work and its supervision gain from the consultation.
- A school invites a psychologist to take a staff group to enhance teachers' confidence and skills in handling disruptive pupils.
- A college of further education asks a counsellor to meet a group of its staff to discuss how to develop their skills in helping with students' problems.
- An organisation feels it is in difficulties. The staff aren't sure whether it needs advice about its administration, its clientele, its staff training programmes or its current emotional climate. It employs an outside consultant to help it clarify these questions.

These examples illustrate the range of consultative work, which is outlined in Figure 2.2. Despite the diversity there is a common theme: the sharing of ideas and expertise to advance the thinking of the consultees.

However, the very diversity of the work needs some attention, for both practical and theoretical reasons. Consultation may be categorised in various ways:

(1) The aim of the work is sometimes primarily to do with training (with problem-solving as a bonus) or primarily to do with problem-solving (with progress in professional skills as a bonus). This circularity, already referred to, is fundamental to consultation.
(2) The focus of the work may be (a) the people with whom the consultees work i.e. their clients, students or patients; (b) the consultees themselves i.e. their own ideas, approaches, skills etc.; or (c) the group, team or organisation in which they work. As is discussed in Chapter 7, this focus may change during the course of the work.

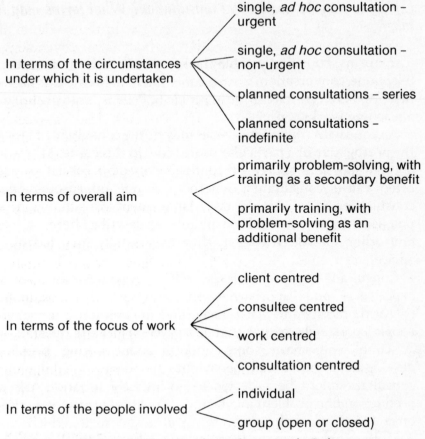

Figure 2.2 Categories of consultative work: outline.

(3) The consultation may be sought to deal with an urgent crisis or it may be a planned piece of work. Similarly it may be an *ad hoc*, one-off occasion; or a planned, single occasion; or an agreed series of meetings.

(4) It may be conducted over the telephone, as a first contact in an emergency might be. Or it may be a meeting at the consultant's or the consultees' place of work. It may involve just consultant and consultee, or a group.

(5) Consultation may be the most appropriate and effective way to bring people with different experience and skills together in a teaching and learning exercise. There need be no particular issue or problem as a focus other than an agreed aim of, say, seeing what architects and psychologists, clergymen and psychiatrists or actors and psychotherapists might learn from each other and develop together.

(2) Who may be involved in consultation? What forms may it take?

The forms consultation may take can therefore include a telephone conversation, a case conference, a planned or *ad hoc* meeting between two or more people (indeed, a large group) or a teaching workshop.

Anyone with consultative skills may be the consultant; it is not the prerogative of a particular profession. In this context there is another possible source of confusion: medical specialists are often called consultants, whether or not interprofessional consultation is what they do. Management consultants may practise interprofessional consultation as described here, or, like any other specialised expert, they may simply give technical advice.

Consultant and consultees will commonly have some experience and approaches in common. For example, psychotherapists and artists may have in common interests in people's personal creativity, while a psychologist and the staff of a school will share some notions about young people's development and social behaviour. In theory a competent consultant might be expected to go into *any* situation (e.g. a production line problem in a factory, a political *impasse* or a crisis on a farm) and help generate an atmosphere in which the consultees (who have the technical expertise) can think through the nature of the problem, clarify it, and draw up the possible options for dealing with it. In practice, however, a reasonable degree of shared understanding of the problem and the situation is helpful.

Sometimes the consultant contributes more than skill in facilitating thought, and there is a real exchange and sharing of expertise. A psychologist may help teachers introduce behavioural approaches in the classroom (Topping, 1986), or a psychiatric team may work out with those referring a patient what the clinicians and the referrers can respectively contribute (Bruggen *et al.*, 1973; Steinberg, 1987, 1988), an approach which I have described elsewhere as a consultative-diagnostic approach, i.e. using two quite different sets of skills (Steinberg, 1983). The consultant does not divest himself of his technical knowledge when entering a consultative relationship, but it takes skill and care to help the consultee make the best use of specific views or methods the consultant may contribute without undermining or replacing the consultee's views and methods.

Where to meet needs a little thought. If you are consulting with the head of a school, meeting in his or her office may be appropriate; on the other hand a meeting with the school staff can be inhibited in such a setting.

Questions like how often the consultative group should meet, for how long, how many meetings there should be, and whether it should be open or closed to new or occasional attenders is open for discussion, but at the earliest possible stage.

Example: A psychologist is asked to provide consultation to a large school for disturbed children, to help the staff manage the children's behaviour. It is agreed that participation will vary, the consultees each time comprising the key staff concerned with the pupils being discussed, plus the head or deputy head of the House. No time limit is set on the work, although it is agreed to review the function and usefulness of the group after one year.

The same psychologist is asked to provide consultation to another school, the purpose being to develop the school along therapeutic community lines. It is agreed that a fixed number of sessions will be held, to fit in with the school's development plans, and that all staff will be invited to attend each meeting.

---

(3) What areas of work are there to be covered in consultation?

There are four main areas, as shown in Figure 2.3.

The relationship between consultant and consultee (A) could be described, for want of better words, as enabling or facilitating. The interchange has been described by Caplan (1970) as coordinate interdependence, because the consultant is as much in need of the consultee's information about the latter's work and role, as the consultee is in need of the consultant's efforts to clarify the questions and the answers. The consultee educates the consultant (Caplan, 1970). See Chapter 8 for a further discussion of this relationship.

The client's relationship with the consultee (B) may be clinical or otherwise therapeutic, or the work may not involve a clientele at all. In a school, the 'clientele' are the pupils.

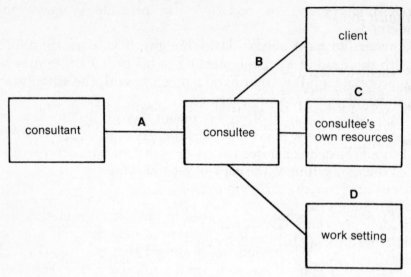

Figure 2.3 Areas of work in consultation.

The consultee's own resources (C) are partly personal and partly professional. Professional resources include technical skill, experience and the other results of past and current training, and in particular the consultee's conceptual models. Personal resources which have a bearing on professional skill include such abilities as the capacity to clarify and solve problems, adaptability, imagination, ability to learn, and fundamental qualities like confidence, intelligence and motivation.

The resources in the work setting (D) are partly those of the working relationships there – the available teaching, supervision and support, the clarity and acceptance of the consultee's role, and the opportunities for collaboration and support; and partly material – time, space, facilities and equipment.

Consultation is largely about helping the consultee to mobilise his or her resources, and these four areas represent the resources. Consultation may pay attention to such things as confidence, problem-solving skills and so on, but it is also important to consider the more basic tools with which work is done. Does the person who is stuck with a work problem have proper training, facilities and supervision? Is the nature of the consultee's job clear and agreed? Does the consultee have an adequate room and a sensible timetable? As we will see later, it is not unusual for what seems like a most complex problem to be resolved by attention to relatively mundane matters.

Which focus?

Consultative work can be classified as:

- client-focussed or centred;
- consultee-focussed or centred;
- work-focussed or centred: i.e. about staff, organisation, programme or curriculum development;
- consultation centred: as needed, to keep the work on course.

What is wanted will usually be agreed clearly from the start; for example, an organisation wanting to introduce a new system of teaching or clinical work will not expect the consultation to become preoccupied with a particular client. If there did seem to be a need for a change of focus then this would ordinarily be discussed and agreed at a meeting designated specifically for reviewing plans.

In practice things are not usually so watertight, because whichever focus is taken, aspects of the others are likely to emerge from time to time. Reasonable focus is maintained by using material from the other three areas as information, as examples of what is happening, and not as the area within which change and development is wanted.

Consultation about individual or team professional skills is relatively easy to keep on task. Client-centred work, however, is likely to lead the consultee to review and reconsider his own style and that of his organisation. In one study of two quite different consultative groups, client-centred work shifted significantly to having work-related matters as the main recurring issue (Steinberg and Hughes, 1987). A shift of focus should be discussed and agreed, rather than just allowed to happen.

Keeping it consultative

If the basics of the consultative approach resolve into three basic questions:

What are you trying to do?
How are you trying to do it?
What's needed for this task?

then it will be clear that the pursuit of these questions as a shared enterprise can lead consultant and consultee into complex and sometimes controversial areas.

Suppose it emerges that the consultee is not getting the sort of supervision, support or cooperation from colleagues that should be expected in that type of work, and that this seems to be a factor in the problem? Suppose the consultee isn't up to the job? Such things arise in consultative work, and confront consultant and consultee with challenges no less difficult than complex problems in the consultee's clientele. The consultant, in order to stick with the consultative task, has to tread a careful path in helping the consultee deal with the areas of work referred to in Figure 2.3 without:

(a) Becoming over-concerned with the clinical (or equivalent) details of a client's case, and therefore becoming more of a supervisor or collaborator than consultant. One form this may take is when the consultant tries to understand the *client* in terms of his own preferred conceptual model or framework (e.g. systemic or psychoanalytic) instead of helping the consultee use or develop his own.
(b) Trying to deal with personal or professional difficulties the consultee may appear to have, thereby tending to adopt a teaching, counselling or even psychotherapeutic role at the expense of consultation.
(c) Becoming too concerned and involved with reported shortcomings among the consultee's colleagues and in the organisation, thereby straying into administrative and political issues.

The point is not that the above material, as data, is inadmissible, or that the focus of attention may not shift from time to time. The consultee may make it clear, for example, that reflecting about his own training, or about the way his team works with its clientele or with each other, will help him think through his work with a client. But while the focus of work in a session may legitimately shift, it is important that the consultant's approach remains *consultative*, and does not become intrusive, interpretive, therapeutic, didactic or directive. Similarly it is not the consultant's job to be supportive or reassuring, both of which have connotations of unconditional backing.

The consultation needs to move forward, illuminating what is going on, but it is up to the consultee what he pays attention to, and what decisions he makes as a result.

To stretch the analogy further, the colour of the illumination matters as much as its direction; you can see quite different things in different lighting conditions. The personnel expert, the psychoanalyst, the family systems therapist, the anthropologist, the sociologist and the political activist of any shade will see a given situation from quite different perspectives, and will be likely to have very different views about what is happening and what needs to be done. Just as Caplan (1970) referred to the problems psychoanalysts have in training as consultants, individual psychotherapists and family therapists (Skynner, 1974; Dare, 1985) have described how things can go wrong in consultation (in these cases in schools) when the consultant brings his own conceptual models and preconceptions to the scene, instead of helping the consultee use his own. If the consultee seems not to be seeing all that clearly, the consultant

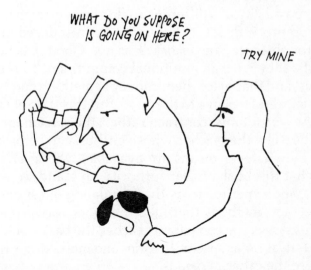

may ask, so to speak, if the consultee has had his eyes tested recently, or perhaps needs a new pair of spectacles; what the consultant does not do is proffer his own to try.

Super Vision

Supervision, conveniently, can have two meanings. There is the supervision of the person overhead, 'overseeing' the work, which is supervision in the hierarchical sense as discussed in

Chapter 1, and there is supervision as used in training, where the work depends on the supervisor's ability to see further, more widely and more clearly than the trainee. In Chapter 1 it was pointed out that while hierarchical supervision is completely distinct from consultation (indeed, perhaps is the most important single distinction to make), training supervision can overlap with it.

Here, then, is an operational problem and potential contradiction at the heart of consultation. The consultant is likely to be interested in the psychology of individuals, relationships and groups, and to have some understanding of the anatomy, social psychology and social dynamics of teams, organisations and other work circumstances. Whether or not the consultant knows more about these subjects than the consultee, it is certainly likely that he or she will be able to see things from an advantageous perspective.

It is this possibility of a different angle of view which helps the consultation proceed; yet it should not be introduced in such a way as to obstruct the *consultee's* view. Good teachers are enthusiasts; they have an emotional commitment to their own perspective, and that helps them convey something composed of facts, ideology and feelings to the pupil. But this style of teaching is not in the consultative contract; rather, the consultant should operate more like the teacher whose enthusiasm is for tackling the issue by whatever means are available, who in effect says let's see what this book or that authority says, and see what we make of it, and experiments with formulating questions, ideas, hypotheses and methods that take the work forward in some way. In this sense, the consultant teaches the basics of scientific thinking; but, as far as specific theories and methods go, he starts from where the other person is.

Psychological exploration in consultation

In Chapter 1 the differences between psychotherapy and counselling on the one hand and consultation on the other were discussed, and the points made that they were as different (and yet with some similarities) as, say, physiotherapy differs from physical education, sports and games. There are some technical (e.g. physiological) similarities between both sorts of activities, but the aims and the personal contracts involved are quite different.

Nevertheless there are times in consultation when consultant and consultee discover that the problem the consultee is having with his client, or with a work problem, appears to reflect a personal conflict. For example, a senior manager may have difficulties in asserting herself appropriately, or a clinician or teacher may find it hard to think straight about a patient or pupil because of personal feelings provoked by the professional relationship. Caplan (1970) referred to this phenomenon as theme interference, and while he considered it to be behind major crises, it was also extremely common in less dramatic forms however healthy and competent the worker or the organisation. Caplan considered anxiety, confusion, muddled and erratic work and repetitive difficulties as indicating theme interference, and noticed stereotyping as a common feature. For example the consultee's conflict may be attributed to the client as an unresolvable problem which has implications for work; he may say 'this sort of family can't be engaged in treatment', 'that sort of problem does badly', or 'our sort of organisation could only work in this way with great difficulty'.

Caplan's advice was that neither consultant nor consultee should focus on the conflict, but on the way the conflict was interfering with the consultee's work. For example, he might put forward approaches or outcomes alternative to the stereotyped outcome the consultee foresees, or introduce for discussion examples that are about other people and occasions, and therefore less laden with feelings and assumptions, but which illustrate similar problems nonetheless. Further, the discussion takes place in a calmer atmosphere, the maintenance of which is part of the consultant's role and skill.

Example: A clinical worker is describing, with evidently mounting tension, the 'impossibility' of a particular patient, and in his heart is foreseeing the breakdown of treatment and the abandonment of the patient who will then commit an offence or get into other serious trouble. His own inclination is to abandon attempts at treatment and treat the problem as something for the social services or the police to respond to.

The consultant accepts that this is one possible outcome, and there are cases where some such step is a reasonable approach to a patient's intractability. He quotes an example or two, preferably known to both of them, where there was just such an outcome, and one or two similar examples where the outcome was different. He encourages the consultee to think with him what can be learned from such examples, about when it is reasonable to terminate treatment, when it is reasonable to carry on, and when it seems that the treatment approach should be modified. How much should we be guided by this sort of information, and how much should we be guided by 'gut feelings'? How do we decide when one should override the other?

Notes

(i)   It is important that the conversation should not become a confrontation, in which the consultant, comfortably uninvolved, either negates the consultee's feelings or treats them as if neurotic, or proceeds to attack his feelings with a 'fire extinguisher' of cold facts and figures. If the consultant concludes that in a problem like this the consultee is merely thinking irrationally, then the consultant, in trying to proceed without understanding the whole of the consultee's predicament, is also acting with inadequate knowledge, and we are left with the blind leading the blind. The consultant has to use empathic and intuitive skills in a friendly and uncritical way, standing as it were beside the consultee and looking at the problem together, rather than challenging the consultee over who has the better way of looking at it.

(ii) Correspondingly, praise is generally as inappropriate in consultation as criticism.

(iii) Having said this, it is common for the consultant to tend to use approaches derived from psychotherapy experience, or to imply praise or criticism as if conducting supervision. Alertness to these deviations is the best way to avoid them.

(iv) A consultee may realise that he or she is indeed in a state of very strong feeling or conflict about a client or a development at work, despite the consultant's efforts to widen the range of thinking and feeling about it. How to continue working effectively despite intrusive and unhelpful feelings can then be a new focus of consultation for a time. Making the focus of work that which was hitherto seen as a peripheral problem is a useful strategy in crises (Steinberg,

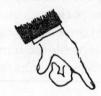
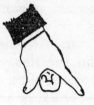

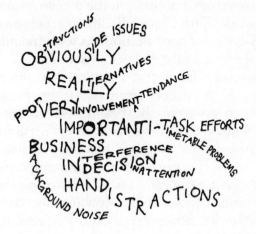

1 SIDE ISSUES
2 OVER-INVOLVEMENT
3 POOR ATTENDANCE
4 TIMETABLE PROBLEMS
5 INTERFERENCE
6 INDECISION
7 INATTENTION
8 BACKGROUND NOISE
9 ALTERNATIVES
10 DISTRACTIONS
11 BUSINESS
12 ANTI-TASK EFFORTS
13 OBSTRUCTIONS
14

1987, 1988), but consultant and consultee should also know when to stop. The consultee who sees that he cannot work effectively because of a personal conflict that he cannot for the moment resolve, should consider (a) working differently, (b) handing over the work to someone else, or (c) getting appropriate counselling or psychotherapy. The latter may be a purely personal decision, but (a) or (b) would need discussing with his supervisor.

The issue of addressing psychodynamic issues without getting into psychotherapy is paralleled by the issue of avoiding supervision. Suppose the consultee, despite or – more likely – because he is so conflict-free and happy-go-lucky, is battling along undertaking work with his client (psychotherapy, sex counselling, or whatever) for which his experience, skill or training is manifestly inadequate? Again, the consultant's task is to help him see this, and to come to a sensible conclusion equivalent to one of the above alternatives, namely to change or give up that work, or seek training in it.

Suppose the conflict-laden or incompetent consultee insists on pressing on? This is discussed in Chapter 7 on the problems and ethics of consultative work. These are all difficult personal issues, and part of the challenge of consultation. As with Income Tax, they may legitimately be avoided but not evaded.

Psychodynamic processes like transference, counter-transference and resistance occur in consultation as in any other relationship, and have been discussed by Berlin (1965). They need handling in a way similar to dealing with other intrusive themes, widening the consultee's thinking and feeling away from the intensely personal. Progress in psychotherapeutic work often requires drawing personal conclusions from the patient's generalisations and allusions. When consultation runs into emotionally-laden obstacles, however, work is advanced by making general observations out of the personal.

To make a perhaps obvious point, consultation requires training, because of the difficulties described above and for the other skills needed. The consultant in training should take his or her work to a supervisor, or, when more experienced, to what is often called peer group supervision; which I think is, by definition, itself consultation.

A theoretical model for consultative work

The worker who begins to move in circles where consultation is studied and practised will soon discover three very different schools of thought, although at present the differences tend to be noted rather than worked with.

One takes for granted that the insights of individual and group dynamic theory, whether in terms of unconscious motivation or systems theory, is as applicable to work problems and their resolution as to any other hitch or difficulty in life. Accordingly, those who take this view adapt their experience of counselling or psychotherapy to their consultative work. On the whole they avoid diagnosing or interpreting their consultees, at least consciously, and in general would accept the basic approach taken in these pages, namely that the material of consultation is what people do rather than why they do it. Indeed they would perhaps be a little hurt if accused of 'therapising' their colleagues, a pertinent if ungrammatical allegation. Nevertheless the theoretical assumptions and professional tendencies may be there.

At least they are likely to avoid assiduously the jargon of psychoanalysis or systems theory, which is more than can be said for the school that has grown out of management theory. Here

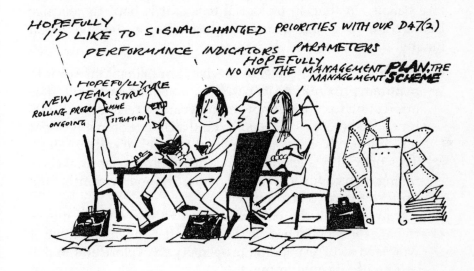

I must reveal my own innocence about a perspective that seems to me to be drawn from a world of drawing boards, flowcharts and notions of group relations that seem based on hierarchical titles (characteristically changed frequently) and job descriptions (usually several dozen items long). The talk in these circles is as cruelly portrayed in the drawing. However, it is to the credit of this approach that it attempts to cope with matters as essential to consultative work as people's feelings and relationships: namely who is trying to do what, with what authority, with what resources (and how do *they* get there), and how do results match intentions?

Some of the concepts discussed by John Bowlby and his colleagues under the general rubric of attachment theory (e.g.

see Bowlby, 1960, 1973, 1980; Heard, 1974, 1978) provide a conceptual model for relationships that is of interest for consultative work in that it allows for both observable social behaviour and presumed intrapsychic processes, and can therefore straddle the worlds of unconscious motivation and objective work and efforts.

It is important to appreciate that the field of attachment has grown out of studies of infant-parent relationships, and the implications for adult relationships are neither clear nor proven. However, it lends itself to the following model, which may be of heuristic value.

It is based on four principal propositions, which have a certain face validity in that, in biological terms, it is hard to conceive human life surviving if any of these propensities were not innate.

(1) Proximity-maintenance: to survive, a human infant needs to maintain proximity to its parent or an equivalent adult. (It is interesting to consider how many years of reliance on adults is needed before a child could stand a chance of independent physical survival: seven years? eight? nine? or rather more?)

(2) This proximity-seeking behaviour requires reciprocal care-taking behaviour from the adult, if food, warmth, and protection are to be provided.

(3) Assuming that the child will need to make some moves towards independence of the above dependent position, it will need a corresponding propensity to explore and in due course use its environment.

(4) To explore and use the environment, the child would need to develop an internal working model comprising an accurate enough picture of the outside world and a sense of its own needs, wishes and capabilities.

Development requires these tendencies to operate together in a dynamic system shown in the diagram. The system is dynamic because each component is interdependent, because the operation of each component requires the operation of the rest of the system, and because each component operates not on an all-or-none basis but as the outcome of one 'move' balanced against another. For example, the child could not explore if the parent's care-taking was fixed: instead, the parent modulates the degree to which exploration is permitted in the light of its parenting skill.

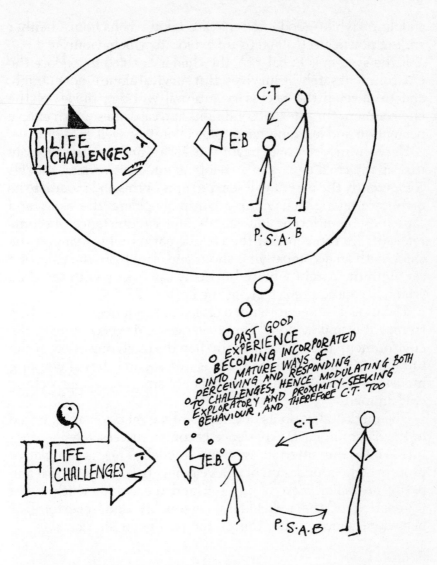

It could be overprotective or underprotective. Correspondingly, the child could be hyper-exploratory or clinging, and becomes a competent explorer if it gets a reasonable balance between exploring and proximity-seeking.

A key control of the system is that exploratory behaviour (EB in the diagram) is necessarily antithetical to proximity-seeking attachment behaviour (PSAB). The child cannot explore and cling at the same time. The more EB, the less PSAB, and vice versa. In cybernetic terms, PSAB steps up care-taking behaviour (CT) (e.g. crying and raised arms promotes picking-up and cuddling) while good-enough care-taking behaviour (neither stifling nor neglectful) steps up exploratory behaviour.

If the system is in balance, the child is enabled to explore the environment safely; it survives. But survival alone is not enough, and to develop the necessary internal working model of the environment the internal conditions and capacities which enable perception and learning need to be operating well enough.

Here the model moves beyond its basics, and we can speculate that as the child begins to develop its internal working models competently the parent will see the signs of this and modulate its own care-taking behaviour accordingly. Here the skills and capacities of different individuals and circumstances become relevant; we can contrast the chaotic parent who snatches the child (with an accompanying shout and slap) from the path of a car, with the parent who unhurriedly catches up with the child who has paused predictably at the kerb.

The model is therefore not a closed one, but open to variables from within and without. The challenges and expectations of the environment (E) may be no more than the inhibiting effect of the unfamiliar (that for which there is not yet an internal working model); or it may be a major provoker of anxiety (an approaching wild animal).

The model takes on its developmental dimension as indicated in the diagram. Each experience becomes successively incorporated into the internal working model. This accumulative process is the foundation of a developing, partly provisional and partly prevailing view of the self and the world which is the foundation of the individual's personality and repertoire of behaviour: among other things, the way he or she copes.

From dependence to consultation

So far the account is of an interactive parent-child model for development and maturation, the internal working models basic ones (e.g. the roadside kerb as marking a safe boundary), and the environmental challenges fairly primitive sources of fear and danger. Further, the underlying theme is of dependence, albeit gradually diminishing dependence.

What reasons may justify the leap from a model of child-parent interaction and development to consultative relationships between adults?

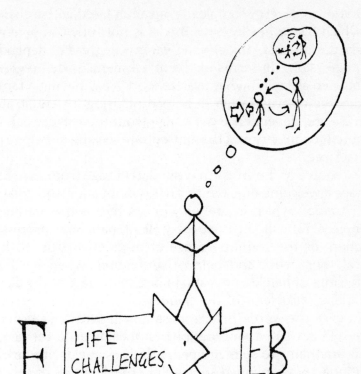

WITH ACCUMULATED EXPERIENCE,
INDIVIDUAL BECOMES SELF-SUPPORTING,
WHICH INCLUDES CAPACITY TO SEEK,
RECOGNISE AND USE HELP ON A
MATURE PEER-PEER BASIS

First, there is no evidence of a fundamental metamorphosis between childhood and adulthood. The process of maturation is a slowly progressive one, with both grown-up and childlike characteristics commonly found on either side of adolescence.

Second, dependent and independent characteristics vary with the environmental challenge. Consider, for example, young children on a ski-slope, confidently handling themselves and their environment, while the adult novice steps carefully, like a baby, holding on tight.

At another level of complexity, an adult faced with a challenge for which his or her internal model is not fully competent can experience distress, anxiety and various degrees of dependence and regression. (In terms of the attachment model, regression can be seen as trying what used to work – e.g. having a tantrum in the face of frustration – instead of using a new strategy.) Distress and dependence can range from the mature acknowledgement of anxiety and the appropriate seeking of help to panic and collapse.

The source of the stress may similarly range from a challenge, perhaps a welcome one, which invites innovation and creativity, to a situation which in one way or another is threatening; for example, a difficult and disturbing client, patient or professional situation, or the common cause of disquiet or distress in the clinical, therapeutic and 'helping' professions when the worker has feelings of helplessness and failure in the face of the distress, demands or problems of the clientele.

But even the words 'helplessness' and 'failure' are emotionally loaded. They carry a connotation of not being up to the task, and this is anathema to so many people in these fields of work. The traditional tough-minded approach to the demands of this work has severe limitations, although it has its strengths too, and these perhaps have been underestimated by the school which favours emotional disclosure all round. The problem is that the

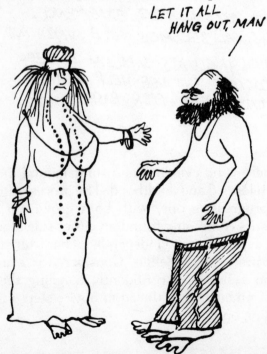

latter approach, supported by the traditionally psychoanalytically orientated and the newer humanistic-radical psychologists alike, takes the perspective that we are all more or less neurotic or misguided, clients and professionals alike, and need to acknowledge this to the professional high priests as a precondition of effective work.

A fundamental mental shift is needed to grasp that in that work which helps workers work effectively, the aim is not to deal with neurosis and incompetence but with training in the emotional and intellectual capacity to do the job. (As has already been pointed out, should neurosis or incompetence emerge then that is not something for the consultation to handle; that is for another time and place.)

Consultation is concerned with the recognition and encouragement of strengths and skills. If we apply to it the attachment model, it represents that development when skilled parenting is replaced by the mature peer-peer relationship. Correspondingly, the unhelpful and inappropriate assumption of the professional worker's helplessness and vulnerability is replaced by appreciation that the demands of many people's work are so great, sometimes unreasonably so, that special strategies and greater than normal resilience are called for.

But all these things are relative, as happens in dynamic situations, and the art and science of consultation is to find the right point of balance. The distance between consultant and consultee has to be right, in several metaphorical senses as well as literally. The balance between being supportive or therapeutic on the one hand and letting consultees go their own way on the other, has to be achieved at a locus which is different from either of these things. The composition of information and techniques needs to be the right mix between those of the consultee and those of the consultant: ideally the latter's contribution to the recipe should be the seasoning rather than the main ingredients. But the ultimate test of consultation, that which marks out its difference from superficially similar activities, is that the consultee helps the consultant to get the balance right.

Summary and concluding note

In Chapter 1 consultation was defined as a joint method of

enquiry in which the consultee is helped to use his own approaches to the full so as to continue working with his own problems and clientele.

In this chapter we have considered in outline the different types of setting and circumstances in which consultation might be sought, and the different types of reasons for seeking it, from crisis intervention to seeking help with a training programme or an aspect of organisational development. In these different situations the common thread is not in the type of problem, but in the type of help sought: not for someone else to take over the problem and tell the consultee what to do, but for joint exploration and experimentation. The consultant does not therefore do something technically specialised on the consultee's behalf, but helps the consultee in what is essentially a problem-solving and educational exercise.

The education is primarily in the systematic approach to problems rather than in a specialised psychological method, and the ideas applied to the problem are, as far as is helpful, those of the consultee. Nevertheless, the consultant as well as consultee brings ideas, past experience and personal perspectives to the consultation, and an essential part of the consultant's skill is to bring these in to help widen the consultee's potential repertoire, without imposing his or her own values and preferences on the consultee's work.

To attempt to sum up the consultative process itself as concisely as possible: the aim is to develop a working relationship and frame of mind in which the components of a problem or issue can be seen as clearly as possible and from a wider perspective, and its requirements sorted into manageable bits and put in order of priority.

Stated more informally, the aim is to help the consultee stand back from the task and, less hampered by over-involvement and tension, to think more clearly and use to the full his or her imagination and capacity for inventiveness and good management.

It is suggested that aspects of attachment theory can throw light on the process by which one person can help another deal with tricky expectations, whether the situation being addressed is an unwelcome difficulty or the challenge of innovation and experiment.

Chapter 3

From Theory to Practice: A Model for Consultative Work

Some rules and guidelines

In this chapter a procedure will be outlined for consultative work, so that the points made in previous pages can be put into practice systematically.

First, to summarise the story so far:

(1) The consultant's job is to help the consultee do his, not to do it for him.

(2) The *aim* of consultative work may be to do with achieving something for his client, or for his work setting or professional programme. Whichever it is, the consultee should also gain in terms of training and professional development.

(3) Sometimes the consultee's professional training and development is the *primary* aim.

(4) Whatever the primary aim, the *focus* of work may be the client, the work or the consultee. The focus may shift from time to time, but the aim should not change without this being made explicit and agreed.

(5) Whatever the aim and the focus, the *process* should remain consultative. Consultation is a peer-peer exercise, so it is the responsibility of consultee no less than consultant to keep the work consultative and not, for example, psychotherapeutic or supervisory.

(6) A decision that something other than consultation is needed, as well as or instead of the consultative work, is not merely a legitimate outcome but, assuming that it is appropriate,

evidence that the consultation is getting somewhere.

(7) There are important expectations of the consultee as well as of the consultant. The consultant has to assume that the consultee is responsible and professionally competent within the normal limitations of his or her position and seniority. The aims of the consultation therefore need to be within the present potential of the consultee.

(8) The aims therefore should be clear and agreed, the focus may shift from time to time as appropriate, while the process remains consultative. The methods of working vary with preference, circumstances and practicality. Some different styles of consultative work are illustrated in the examples in Chapters 4–6.

First contact

Consultation is sometimes initiated by the consultant. For example, a patient is referred by telephone to a psychiatrist, and the latter suggests discussing the situation rather than simply sending an appointment. This conversation may turn into a consultation, or a time may be arranged for the involved professional workers to meet. This may be the only meeting anticipated, and the sequence outlined in Figure 3.1 for a series of meetings can be condensed and adapted for the purposes of a single session.

Alternatively, a complicated situation may be perceived, with a certain amount of uncertainty and confusion about who wants what. The example given in the first chapter would have come into this category. In this case the consultant should suggest a preliminary meeting with the necessary people present. These are the people either whose presence is required for progress to be made, or who, though not participating themselves, are prepared to ensure that there is agreement about how the consultation will be used.

An independent, autonomous worker can of course make these decisions for himself or herself. But autonomy is not invariably clear.

(1) First contact.
(2) Preliminary consultation:

- who to meet initially: managers, unless consultee is autonomous
- aims of the person or organisation
- general aims for the consultation
- confirmation that consultation is needed
- who to meet in the consultative work, if different from above
- practicalities – timetabling, etc.

(3) As above – but now with the agreed consultees
(4) Working:

- getting to know the consultees
- getting to know their organisation
- clarifying the issues or problems
- clarifying resources (individual, work setting) available
- working with matching resources to problems (e.g. what done so far, shortfalls, things learned, problems remaining, new issues identified)
- sorting work into manageable pieces and acceptable priorities
- attention to the working methods within the consultation; review if necessary

(5) Review of progress of the consultation and next steps
(6) Ending

Figure 3.1 An outline schema for consultative work.

The preliminary consultation

This meeting is very commonly omitted, so that essential preliminaries are either never cleared up satisfactorily, or emerge distractingly later, e.g. at the first consultation proper.

The meeting needs in some way to include the views of those authorising consultation (e.g. the senior managers) and the consultees. Sometimes both meetings consist of the same people; sometimes the meeting is one in which some senior managers and some consultees participate; and sometimes the first contact with senior managers will have dealt with the formalities, and the rest is delegated to the consultees. Whether or not payment is an issue, it should be quite clear who is employing you and on what basis.

The following need establishing, at the first contact or at the preliminary consultation, if not both:

(i)   Brief mutual introductions are important; note that you may well not immediately remember people's names and roles. If this is likely to be a problem, e.g. in a large and changing group with complicated duty rotas and hierarchies, a written out list may help. Make a mental note that this is also an early example of how the place and the people operate.

(ii) Discuss what is expected of the consultation to come. If this is not yet clear or generally agreed, as is often the case, this becomes one of the focuses for consultation. (For example, it is reasonable to offer consultation to sort out uncertainties about whether consultation is actually needed.) Early on you will detect 'unofficial' as well as formal hierarchies in the group. Check that everyone agrees with the views of those who are most forthcoming, or at least are happy to let them take a lead. Again, this will be a characteristic of the group and their work outside the group, and a factor to be worked with.

(iii) Explain what you have to offer, i.e. your own approach to consultative work. See if it is acceptable. If not, discuss what adaptations are wanted and feasible. A group might want occasional sessions in which you conduct a teaching session on a relevant topic. I would hesitate to intersperse consultative meetings with formal lectures, but teaching can be conducted on consultative lines, as mentioned in Chapter 1. In other words, it is important to be willing to negotiate to see how your consultative skills and interests can be matched to what is wanted.

(iv) Discuss when and where to meet, how long each meeting should take, and over what period of time. My own preference is for meeting regularly and sticking firmly to starting and stopping times. Discuss whether there will be occasional meetings specifically to review progress.

(v)   Will you work by yourself, or arrange for your own supervision of your work? If so, you should let the consultees know, pointing out that it is you who are being overseen, not them. Nevertheless, confidentiality is still an issue and this, too, needs discussion.

(vi) Will the sessions be recorded in any way? Notes are helpful in several ways, and in addition may be material for research, in which case you will already have consulted an appropriate person about how best to keep notes. The minimal record I keep is a dated sheet listing who was present and the main themes that emerged.

Reflection about what you are getting into

An aspect of record-keeping that is more for yourself is that your professional base, especially if a hospital, may not officially recognise consultative work, and have no official way of recording it. It would, for example, be wrong to record consultative work under the name of a client about whom consultation is taking place, unless he or she was already a patient of your Department.

Further thoughts will be about how to proceed, but if there are remaining doubts or uncertainties then consult someone, for example the consultees. The essence of consultation is that every doubt or lack of clarity to do with starting, proceeding or finishing is not to be seen as a peripheral nuisance or worry, but as a further focus for consultation.

It is of course essential that your own work contract permits commitment and time to do the work you are planning to undertake. This is particularly true if you are in training. Some consultative work benefits from being long-term, and if it is likely to be interrupted by job changes it is important to foresee this, and to discuss the implications with the consultees.

Beginning
Example

Most of these few pages are about practicalities. It is also important for the consultant to be alert to the undercurrents of feeling and attitude of the group, particularly in this first meeting. Feelings associated with the various possible misunderstandings about the nature of consultation will be around; some caricatures may make the point.

Jack and Jill are already an alliance in the organisation and in the group; there is some institutional history to their expressing discontent about the way the organisation and the seniors have operated, and their concern for the setting up of outside consultation has generated an ambivalent mixture of feelings towards them composed partly of gratitude and partly of irritation. Will the consultation be a success or a waste of time? Will Jack and Jill be affirmed in their wisdom?

Joan has had problems for which she has moved from job to job and therapist to therapist. She is currently attending an alternative healer. She might be leaving soon. She understands that this isn't a therapeutic group but another part of her hopes that getting her colleagues all together (they are otherwise rarely in the same place at the same time) with a wise and caring outsider is going to reveal something helpful and do something supportive and comforting for them all.

Roger has had problems with other people, and has also had a number of jobs. He might be leaving soon. He has seen people like the consultant before, and is sceptical. Being a fair-minded man he has come along willingly, despite having better things to do.

Jeff is new, enthusiastic and willing to learn. The others don't yet know him well.

Jane feels and holds more responsibility. She knows what consultation is. There is a tension in her curiosity about how it is going to go.

The consultant is unaware of all this, but knows that such constituents of the 'background noise' will be influential on the work of the organisation and the group.

Getting started:
(1) Start with mutual introductions, if the group aren't those which were present at the preliminary consultation.
(2) Again, if there are new people, briefly ask what they have heard from senior managers or the other consultees about the consultation. There can still be surprises at this stage, however carefully things have been explained at the preliminary meeting (e.g. 'to teach psychotherapy,' you may be told, or 'a support group'.)
(3) If you are consulting with a group, check that the timing of the meetings and the consultees' timetable, duty rota,

preferences etc. match with the plans made so far. When you hear that it's fine 'but it means the Deputy will only be able to attend on his days off', or someone thirty years in the post 'won't be able to make it but she says never mind' you will again be learning something about how the group or organisation works.

(4) You will now begin to learn about the consultees' reasons for the consultation. How this is conducted is very dependent on personal style, and the examples that follow and the accompanying commentary is only one way of proceeding, and will not meet all situations.

Consider:

The central issue or problem.
  A brief description.
  The consultees' way of handling it so far.
  What's gone right - not so much in terms of the
    client or the situation progressing; rather in terms of how
    far the consultees' strategies so far are achieving what they
    are aiming for.
  In similar terms, what (if anything) has got stuck, could be
    going better, or what (if anything) is going wrong?
  What has helped - in terms of consultees' ideas,
    skills, experience, approach, etc.
    What's not helped enough, in these terms, and
    what would help more?
  What has helped, in terms of collaboration with colleagues,
    supervision and teaching received, the wider administra-
    tion, material resources, organisation, timetabling, etc?
    What's not helped enough, in these terms, and what would
    help more?
  What light does the above shed on:
    The nature of the original issue?
    The way the consultees approach it?
    The way the group, team or organisation works?
  What does this tell us about any changes or alternative
    strategies needed? For example -
    Does the issue or any aspect of it need redefinition?
      Dividing it into a number of sub-tasks for different
      approaches, different people and different timetabling is
      one form of redefinition.

Are some aspects of the task more urgent or easier to deal with than others? What priorities can the different aspects be given? How will that be decided? Does this lead to any new proposals?

Does anything need to be modified, and how much is best left as it is, in the consultees' approach? How will that be decided? How will priorities be decided? Does this lead to any proposals?

Does anything need to be modified, and how much is best left as it is, in the way the larger organisation works? How will that be decided? How will priorities be decided? Does this lead to any proposals?

How will change, stability or stasis be recognised and monitored? How will we know when goals are achieved?

Continuing work

Consultative work then proceeds broadly on the above lines, with review, redefinition and a degree of circularity. The sequence of questions within the meeting to do with

(1) defining the problem,
(2) clarifying resources for handling aspects of it,
(3) considering and reconsidering resources, and
(4) considering and reconsidering strategies,

moves on to working with how the issue or problem is currently being handled in day-to-day work, and brings back to the consultation

(1) how the problem has been resolved or the issue handled, and
(2) what if anything still requires to be dealt with; hence a further definition of the issue or problem.

Keeping to the task requires that consultant and consultees keep in sight the purpose of their meeting. Other sorts of activities may be thrown up by the consultative work, e.g. someone may want further training, another may want personal counselling, someone may want to challenge the senior management or reorganise the duty rota, or someone else may want the client to be seen by a specialist. Such questions are for final decision and action outside the consultative meetings.

Methods

Imagination will be needed to adapt the above sequence to all the very varied circumstances of consultation, from a twenty minute telephone discussion of a caller's problem to several years' regular consultative work with an organisation. Sometimes consultation is helped by holding an all-day or weekend meeting. Nevertheless, there is the common thread throughout:

- What are you trying to do?
- How are you trying to do it?
- What are you learning as a result?

The style of the consultation will also vary with the participants, but in my view it should be conversational and questioning. To an outsider, it should sound like a discussion between peers, not like a clinical history-taking. Still less should it be like a psychotherapeutic session with the consultee conducting a monologue interspersed by an occasional 'uh-huh' from the consultant. Caplan (1970) has warned of the uselessness of a consultation consisting of a long account by the consultee to a silently listening consultant, who at the end is asked 'So what shall I do?' In my experience this can be a rude awakening.

The consultant should try to avoid offering reassurance or 'support'; one carries the connotation that the consultant knows what's best, the other implies general encouragement for whatever the consultee wants to do. Consultation functions between these two points, as a shared critical appraisal and reappraisal of what the consultee is attempting, and neither reassurance nor support is appropriate. When the consultant finds himself doing this, he should consider, perhaps with the consultee's help, whether they are straying off the task.

It is also in the spirit of consultation (i.e. that neither consultant nor consultee know everything nor nothing) that the consultant's remarks aren't too challenging, directive or negative. My advice is to frame comments as questions whenever possible. For example, instead of: 'You'll never manage to keep a behaviour programme going with so many staff coming and going all the time', ask 'How will you keep a behaviour programme going consistently?'

For similar reasons the consultant's doubts about the consultee's approach can often be put positively, and in a way that encourages thought (on both sides). For example, instead of: 'I think it will cause problems if you see your client on demand instead of regularly', ask 'What are the advantages and disadvantages of doing it that way?'

Consultation consists mostly of talking, but supplementary techniques can be useful. In trying to grasp the complexities of

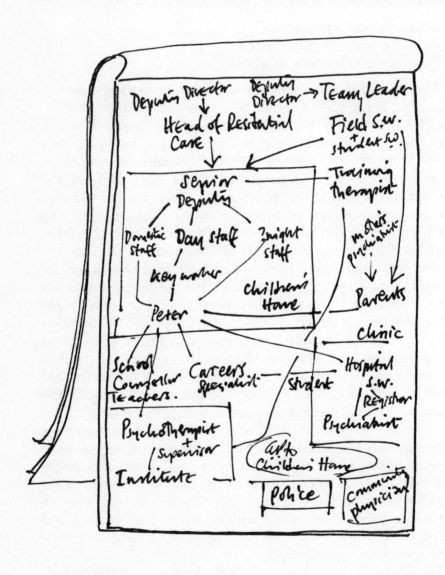

Connections: pre-clarification.

organisations, I find it helps to use a blackboard or flip chart to draw a diagram of people, departments and connections. Sculpting techniques and role play can be helpful, but require experience of these approaches, and particular vigilance that the purpose is clear and stays on task: i.e. as an aid to understanding the components of a work issue or problem. Such periods within a consultative session need clear and formal demarcation from the discussion leading up to it and the drawing of conclusions that follows.

To take some simple examples of creative and action techniques in consultation:

- The consultees may be considering problems arising during the admission of a new young person to a children's home, and feel it would be helpful to look in some depth at the tensions and disruptions that occur. This can be explored using role play, with careful attention to structuring the session and 'de-roling' after it.

- The way a multidisciplinary team is organised may be causing confusion, with muddle about who is in charge of which groups of people, who collaborates most closely with whom, where the most support comes from, and so on. Sculpting the situation can clarify relationships, and a further sculpt of what would improve things (from the points of view of different people) can be illuminating. (Sculpting involves people placing themselves in a space and in relation to other people in a way that conveys in three-dimensional terms how a situation seems and feels. It includes choice of posture too, e.g. looking towards or away from someone else, or being on a pedestal (literally, in the sculpt) or on the floor.)

- A consultative group may feel that discussion doesn't convey sufficiently how each sees the other's role. The consultant suggests that each draws a simple coat of arms depicting how they see their own function, and that of a colleague. A senior member draws hers in terms of feeding bottles and cots, with

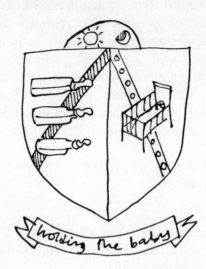

'holding the baby' as a motto. A colleague's drawing of her is of someone behind a desk, dealing with paperwork and telephones and with 'do not disturb' as the motto.

Creative and activity techniques are most likely to be appropriate when professional and organisational development is the primary focus of work, but there is no reason why they may not have a place in client-centred work too. For an account of these techniques in general see for example Jennings (1985, 1986).

Reviewing overall direction and purpose

Consultation can clearly be amusing and diverting, and it is important to check, preferably at specially designated meetings, how far it is achieving what it set out to achieve when work began. The questioning applied to the primary task can be applied no less rigorously to the consultation itself, with questions raised about its usefulness and methods. If appropriate, new goals can be set, or the decision made to bring the sessions to an end.

Ending

This needs a little attention, because any group that has met over time will have generated feelings and relationships and ending will leave a gap, particularly if the members have come together from elsewhere. This should be acknowledged, and the implications for work continuing without the consultative meetings acknowledged. It is worth reviewing how the consultee's own work might change, if at all, particularly in relation to colleagues who have not been participants.

Variations on this scheme

The introduction of active and creative methods (if the consultees want them) is not too great a departure from the principle of using the consultee's own concepts and methods, because creative techniques are by their nature facilitatory and exploratory rather than didactic. A sculpt (see above) of a working situation will stimulate in different consultees their own ways of seeing an issue and acting on it, no less than can discussion. Moreover it widens the consultee's skills in problem-assessing and problem-solving, which again is part of the consultative task. Lyons *et al.* (1987) have described one way among many for creative therapists to work on a consultative basis, in this case in the field of special education.

The introduction of formal teaching, i.e. setting out to convey new ideas and new skills to the consultees, does challenge the definition given earlier (i.e. to make the most of the skills the consultees already have). Dare (1982) points out that it is hard to envisage consultation as completely devoid of imparting information about, for example, child development or managing clients' behaviour according to principles developed in behavioural science. Thus some authorities distinguish *behavioural consultation*, where the consultant takes an active, directive role and shows careworkers and teachers how to use behavioural approaches in their settings, from the type of consultation described so far in this book. (For example, see Tharp and Wetzel, 1969; Yule *et al.*, 1977, Gallessich, 1982; Conoley and Conoley, 1982; Topping, 1986; Kolvin *et al.*, 1981; Lane, 1986; Tattum, 1986.)

I believe it is worth recognising the distinctive qualities of behavioural consultation, but there is no reason to exclude direct behavioural or any other teaching from any form of consultative work if (a) it is clearly seen to be within the consultation contract and related to the original and agreed aims; (b) that the consultees want it, and see what is learned as becoming part of their own repertoire of skills, and appropriately so; and (c) the work with the clientele is carried out by the consultees. With these provisos, I do not think the essence of the consultative approach is undermined.

What I have described elsewhere as a *consultative-diagnostic approach* (Steinberg, 1983, 1987, 1988) is not a dilution or variant of consultation but a deliberate attempt to bring two quite distinct approaches to bear on a single problem, to help share work between groups of people who need to be involved and collaborating. The diagnostic approach, which is central to the medical model of working (the 'medical model') is quite distinct from the consultative model. The essence of the diagnostic (medical) model is not to do with supposed physical causes, but concerned instead with the notion that the individual has something 'wrong' within, a disorder, be it in behavioural, psychodynamic or biological terms. The diagnostician assesses this in terms of symptoms and signs – what the patient reports, how he or she behaves, and so on – and goes on to match what is seen to specialised conceptual frames of reference (e.g. neurochemical functioning, behaviour theory, psychodynamic theory). The psychoanalyst and the behavioural psychologist do this no less than does the physician (Tyrer and Steinberg, 1987).

The consultative approach is quite different, being concerned not with diagnosis, but with the description of problems in the language and concepts of the consultee. The consultee's concepts, and methods, may be biological, behavioural, psychodynamic, educational-developmental, to do with child care, or simply about how people generally carry on.

There are many problems, especially in the psychiatric and social work fields, where the person referring a client for help is stuck, and there may well be a use for (say) psychiatric, psychotherapeutic or other psychological intervention, but there is still much that the original referrer could, and would want, to contribute. A purely consultative approach would play down the specialist contribution, while a traditional diagnostic approach could undermine the work the referrer is already doing.

In such circumstances, clarified and agreed at the first contact, the specialist can see the client for either a limited or extended assessment, and then go on to hold a consultative session with those already involved in the client's care. In this consultation the question is about the respective contributions of all concerned – including, of course, the specialist – to the client's care, and how they will jointly collaborate and monitor progress. By thinking of this specifically as a joint consultative-diagnostic approach the advantages of both types of work are sustained.

Summary and concluding note

In this chapter some basic guidelines to consultative work have been developed into a general schema. However, although there is a consistent theme to consultative work it is adaptable to many different settings and situations. Consultation may be undertaken as a fairly short conversation on the telephone about the caller's client, as a single case conference about a patient's case, as a series of meetings aimed at helping staff and organisation development, or as a meeting planned to last all day or for several days. The schema can be adapted to all these circumstances and settings with a little imagination. Variations on the basic schema are introduced, when it is appropriate to bring in the technical skills of the consultant in parallel with his or her consultative function.

Examples are given of using creative techniques in the consultative work itself, of teaching about behavioural approaches, and of introducing clinical diagnostic approaches in special circumstances as a complement to consultation.

Chapter 4

Consultation in Practice I: Examples from Different Settings

Introduction

This and the next two chapters will examine consultation adapted to different settings and circumstances.

One of the distinctions already drawn is between consultation in crisis intervention or problem-solving on the one hand, and consultative approaches to new developments in working and training on the other. There is no denying the feelings of anxiety and helplessness that can be around in the former situation, in contrast with the confidence and optimism associated with the latter. The fantasies about the one are to do with weakness, failure and being rescued (feelings that the consultant may unwittingly reinforce), while the other type of situation is seen as positive, creative and forward looking. It is the difference, in fantasy, between being helped out of a hole and being helped up a ladder.

As far as the consultative process is concerned this distinction is not important, although of course the respective feelings need to be attended to whatever they happen to be. The point is that anxiety and guilt is common among the 'helping' professions and can go very deep. Bennet (1979, 1987) and Balint (1968) have discussed these and other feelings that get in the way of healthy functioning and work in relation to medical practice, and Menzies (1970, 1974) in relation to nurses in large institutions. The literature on counter-transference in psychotherapy represents another way into the complex field of professionals' feelings (e.g. see Sandler, Dare and Holder, 1970; Sandler 1976; Brown and Pedder, 1979). The artist, the engineer, the soldier, the scientist and the lawyer tend to take the challenging aspect of their work as a matter of course; other professionals' work is by no means free of feelings, and sometimes very strong feelings, but there does not seem to be the same burden of guilt experienced by the 'helpers and carers' who, the consultant will find, quite often are conscious of falling short, being found wanting, and so on; the disabling influence of a preoccupation with repercussions, whose source may be within or without.

The consultant should pay attention to whatever is constructive and creative in all situations, the team crisis no less than the team seeking consultation about an exciting new development, and should try to help the consultees see this too.

The consultant will find that as well as needing some understanding of the psychology of group and individual functioning, another 'map' is needed: a guide to the anatomy and operations of organisations, and those aspects of management that straddle psychology and sociology. This too is a big subject, and it is only possible here to draw the aspiring consultant's attention to the fact that the subject exists, that it has a vast literature and more than its fair share of jargon, controversy and waffle; a point made only to ensure that the newcomer, reeling from the highways and byways of psychology, does not make the mistake of thinking that the first account of 'the organisation' he comes across necessarily contains the truth.

In a helpful short introduction, Ryle (1982) picks out some of the factors and components in the functioning of organisations. As a guide to beginning to conceptualise the settings within which people work, consider:

(1) What the organisation actually does. (Thus a hospital, for example, does far more than 'treat the sick'.)
(2) How skills, responsibilities, roles and authority are distributed throughout the organisation, and who deals with which of its various aims.
(3) Where power and control lie in relation to the range of aims and responsibilities.
(4) How decisions are made and authority asserted.
(5) How communications systems operate: who with whom, and about what? What is left out? Who decides? Are there

sub-groups which communicate only within an insulated group?

(6) What value is given to which functions? Who decides?

(7) What conflicts arise in this mesh of different aims, roles and power distribution? How are they dealt with?

(8) What different types of authority are there? Authority may be formal and legal (the general manager), traditional (the doctor), charismatic (a 'character'), or informal ('no one messes with that particular member of the night staff').

(9) To what extent are some of these matters clear (e.g. in an autocracy) or blurred (e.g. in a quasi-democracy)?

(10) How does the organisation relate to other groups and organisations, formally and informally?

In this chapter examples and vignettes will be given to illustrate the guidelines in Chapter 3 and elsewhere. The following settings are used to illustrate the different forms consultation can take, and the wide range of questions that can arise:

(1) A consultative group in a local authority children's home.

(2) A school which has a large number of adolescents with behaviour problems.

(3) A medical ward dealing with severely ill patients.

(4) An in-patient psychiatric unit.

(1) A consultative group in a Local Authority children's home

A psychologist has begun to take a weekly staff consultative group in a children's home.

At one meeting the problem is presented of what to do about mentally handicapped children. Since a nearby hospital unit for the mentally handicapped was closed down, as part of a community-orientated policy, and a home for mentally handicapped young people closed for lack of staff, more such boys and girls were being referred to the home.

The home has one girl, Susan, who is mentally handicapped. But the Local Authority's placement department now wants the home to accept another child whose foster care has broken down because of behaviour problems.

For a time the meeting loses itself in generalisations about

'Them': the Department of Social Services, which makes demands on the home without providing resources, which sends children in at short notice with inadequate preparation, which didn't listen when unspecified people warned against closing down the special home for handicapped children.

The consultant notices also the tendency to stereotype mentally handicapped children: that behaviour problems are to be expected, that they will be hard to handle, that the staff don't have the necessary skills to manage them. She is tempted to draw a parallel between the negative and defensive attitudes of the staff towards the Department and similar feelings about the children being discussed.

A junior member of the group accuses the group of insensitivity and paranoia. The head of the home now joins in, explaining in a reasoned way that they would like to be able to help, but don't have the necessary skills and resources. The junior member of staff becomes quite heated and says this is nonsense, that she has a mentally handicapped sister who is no different from anyone else except being a slow learner, and the head of the home is just prejudiced and over-anxious.

Big issues are coming up. Quite significant personal criticisms are being expressed which touch on the competence of the head of the home, who is perceived to be taking refuge in rationalisation, the Department which is being accused of moving children around like pawns and not caring about staff, and one member of the team is holding forth emotively about her sister. Not far below the surface the consultant believes she detects anxiety and antipathy about mentally handicapped children in general, nicely evaded by virtue of the 'good one' already resident.

The consultant asks about people's experience of mental handicap. What it means, what mental handicap is like, what is and isn't special about relating to people with mental handicap. About half of the group can give personal accounts, and the meeting becomes quite absorbing. No-one points out the striking differences between the handicaps described in the various anecdotes, so the consultant mentions it. They go on to discuss the wide range of different ways of responding to mental handicap, from organising major behavioural treatment programmes at one extreme to, at the other, making no more personal adjustment than one would to any other person.

They now return to the opinion of the head of the home, that they don't have the resources and the training. They now agree that they have what is needed for some young people with mental handicap, but not for others. With the dust somewhat settled, the point made by the head of the home seems reasonable after all: they should perhaps assume that mentally handicapped children being referred to a children's home do need something special, rather than the reverse, and as a team they should be reasonably sure they can meet their needs.

The discussion now moves on to considering what degrees of mental handicap they can manage, which leads to clarification that intellectual handicap and social impairment are different, and that there are many degrees of both. This then leads to consideration of how far it is appropriate to stretch their skills through in-service training to accommodate at least some of the handicapped children referred to them.

The meeting lets go of its negative preoccupation with 'Them' outside. The consultant reminds the meeting of the people concerned with placement in the Department. Does the team want to take their conclusions further, and if so would it want to have some policy discussions with them? The group is interested in doing so. The consultant wonders aloud about the pros and cons of deciding in this meeting, or putting the question on the agenda of the home's administrative meeting. The head of the home thinks it should go to the next administrative meeting, and no one disagrees.

Comments

In this example the consultant has had to make an effort not to let her own views on policy intrude. She felt it was a good thing for a children's home to accept mentally handicapped children, and for a time her feelings included sympathy with the junior member of staff who spoke about her sister, and a little antipathy towards the caution of the head of the home. The group took on a basic assumption that it was 'good' to widen their intake to include handicapped children.

The exploration of such realities in the light of everyone's actual knowledge of mental handicap and its management, and their experience of the people concerned, resulted in a more pragmatic discussion. The group, in its enthusiasm, wanted to make a new policy there and then. The consultant wanted the group to consider the advantages and disadvantages of deciding then and there, and felt the head of home should decide, because the way the team worked was to let him have the last word.

The consultant felt there were two issues left over that she would invite the team to discuss. One was whether they had any observations about the process by which they had reached their tentative proposal. This was because she felt the way discussion had proceeded had something important to teach about how they reached decisions over controversial matters. Second, she had noticed that the group had very nearly decided then and there the team's policy, or made as if to; she would ask the head of home if that was what he wanted, and, further, if he wanted to discuss that with the group. It did seem that in, correctly, going along with the home's formal way of working, it seemed necessary to prompt the head of the home from time to time about his senior role.

Notes

Some aspects of consultation demonstrated in this example include:

(i)   Note that the consultation proceeds with a degree of circularity: the main issue is kept in sight, and is returned to in the light of new information and perspectives and the possibility of reconsidered attitudes and feelings (see Figure 4.1). The circularity, therefore, is one which should leave consultant and consultee better informed and more competent with each completed cycle. The example given here is of a problem which is not far short of a crisis, but the process of widening perspectives to examine alternative ways forward is just as appropriate when the focus of consultation is quite different (for example in developing new training programmes or working methods as described in Chapter 6).

(ii) The move away from heated feelings and anxieties to look at the facts.

(iii) Avoidance of the temptation to go straight into either 'heavy' personal or group dynamic issues, or into policies and politics; but nevertheless drawing attention to the existence

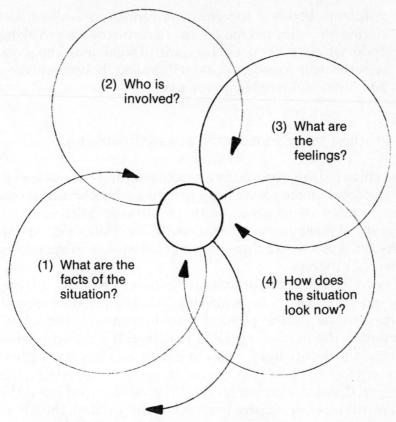

... Continuing reappraisal at a more informed level

Figure 4.1 Circularity in consultation.

of these influential attitudes, and inviting the group to make time to consider them.

(iv) The consultant's sense of balance in deciding what to leave to the group and what to bring to its attention. She was conscious of the group process of blaming, stereotyping and then dismissing the outside world ('Them' in the Department) and brought them back in, so to speak, when the group was ready to discuss outside expectations more realistically. At this point she could have made a comment that the group, having done some work, were now able to look more realistically and positively at the possible role of the people 'outside'.

(v) In a similar vein, helping the group see that there was a difference between the group as ventilator, explorer and clarifier of issues and the group as a formal decision-making body, which it was not. This clarified something about the way the team functioned, as well as about how conclusions and decisions were being reached.

(2) A school for adolescents with behaviour problems

A psychiatrist is approached by a headmaster and a school governor to provide some consultative help to a school which takes a large number of teenagers with problematic behaviour. He suggests a preliminary meeting with the staff, and having started suggests two or three meetings to be followed by an early review of progress.

They all meet in the headmaster's study. The head, a large, jolly and forceful man, sits behind his desk, and introduces people as they trickle in: the physical education master, the school counsellor, the head of maths, a part-time teacher who takes pottery, the deputy head, a parent governor, a biology teacher, the chaplain (part-time) who has an important pastoral role, the technical drawing instructor, one of the welfare workers at the school (the other being part-time and not here today), the school doctor is going to come if he can, the French teacher, the school's nurse, the senior teacher who is also the careers master, and an education welfare officer, one of two who is very involved with the school. There are more teachers to come.

After some mutual introductions, begun again several times as more people squeeze into the room, the consultant asks people to say, briefly, what they would like this meeting to begin to consider. They use a flip-chart to draw up a list. They then draw up a list of what the school already offers, with its various sources of expertise. They talk around these themes, and try to draw up a list of priorities for attention. The consultant also encourages talk about the school's recent history.

The client-centred (i.e. pupil) problems that emerge are a mixture of educational and social disadvantage and poor behaviour, ranging from a lack of social skills to major disruptive and aggressive conduct. The skills available are general teaching and special remedial skills (used effectively), work with parents and families (used well but only patchily) and individual counselling skills (again well conducted, but patchily, by several different professions), and with little liaison with teachers on the one hand or with the family workers on the other. Recreational and creative work is seen as part of the academic curriculum, and without implications for the pupils' behaviour. Behaviour management has been little used. The school had a psychologist in the past who was a skilled individual psychotherapist, and who has not so far been replaced because of uncertainty at headmaster and school governor level about the school's needs and the job description. Financial considerations are thought to have helped this delay to be perpetuated.

The consultant points out what a complex organisation the school is, and, for his own clarity, suggests a further exercise 'on paper', drawing up on a blackboard a diagram of the school hierarchy and who is involved with whom, an exercise which is achieved with much discussion and a great deal of use of the duster.

There is a certain amount of muddle in how the school uses its considerable resources, but it is by no means an institution in a crisis. It does good work with difficult pupils, and has a good reputation, but there was a feeling that it could do more. The consultant suspects something else lies behind this, but puts that question aside for the moment. The first priority is to find out what goes on, the anatomy and physiology of the place so to speak, and anticipating this he had asked in advance for a flip-chart or blackboard to be available. The information gathered comes under the headings

- problems;
- people and skills;
- a diagram of links between personnel.

The group's individual contributions to the diagram proves a challenging but stimulating and amusing exercise, and helps the group work together and use each other's knowledge. There are all sorts of discoveries, for example about how 'part-time' someone is, who is employed by whom, and so on. It also helps people clarify their own roles, and at a future meeting they say so. This leads onto a fuller review of what each person can and cannot do, and therefore the school's capabilities and limitations too.

The group decides at the third meeting that staff skills in

behaviour management techniques could usefully be enhanced, and suggests that consultation about behavioural skills could be a useful component of the psychologist's job description. This frees the headmaster and governor to talk about advertising this post, and the headmaster's impending retirement, and the governors' uncertainty about what new directions the school may take; all this emerges as the hidden item on the agenda.

Comment

The consultant suspected, correctly, that in so complex a set-up the informal authority of many different people – i.e. their personal and professional skills rather than their formal position – would be important here. Nevertheless their individuality could be enabled or undermined depending on their relationship with the formal senior people (head, deputies, governors). Priority was given to finding out who could do what, with the formal hierarchy next on the agenda.

Notes

(i)   The picture the consultant gained at the first meeting, of heterogeneity, much promise and a certain amount of muddle, led him to suggest two or more clarifying meetings to be followed by a review of progress at an earlier stage than usual. This would allow for a change in function of the meeting from problem-sorting and skill-clarifying into the more pupil-focussed working group that appeared to be wanted. Should they meet in the head's study, with him behind the desk? Should it be open to whoever could come, or somewhat more stable in membership? How would they decide? How would views and decisions about the psychologist's post be reached? Is it all right for one governor to participate?

(ii) The possibilities for the group's future, following the review, are open. There may be a place for limited membership groups to take on the task of developing behavioural skills, perhaps with the help of the new psychologist when appointed. There may be room for a regular meeting to co-ordinate counselling and family work with the other activities in the school. But there still seems to be some untackled issues (e.g. the impending period of change) and some untapped skills (e.g. making more of creative work and social skills training) and this group may have a continuing function for a time, up to the second review meeting.

(iii) The idea that a psychologist might teach the staff (or a proportion of them: see Yule *et al.*, 1977) behavioural techniques, rather than carrying out behaviour therapy with selected pupils, was a new one to many of the staff. The consultant introduced the idea for the staff to consider.

(3) A medical ward dealing with severely ill patients

A psychiatrist is asked by a ward sister to provide consultation to a ward which contains a large number of seriously and often terminally ill people. It is busy, crowded, overstretched and is used by several different medical teams. It is a teaching hospital, so that key medical staff (registrars, senior registrars and house officers) are constantly changing. A large proportion of the nursing staff are very junior and in training. Other staff, including physiotherapists and occupational therapists, come and go with little involvement with the nursing team. Morale looks all right, but the psychiatrist gets an impression of a degree of contained distress. For example, the patients are often very worried and unhappy but don't like to trouble the busy doctors and nurses, especially as many of the latter are clearly still in their teens. The ward sister has a clear picture of the situation and gives what support she can to patients and junior nurses, but seems very stretched herself to achieve this and to supervise and co-ordinate the constant flow of activity and technical tasks in the ward. She seems brisk, bright and brittle. There are twenty other wards in a similar position; this is one of the better staffed units.

The psychiatrist decides that the situation looks impossible. Too many things seem unsatisfactory, yet firmly embedded in the way the institution works. He continues in his existing role of seeing patients referred to him from that ward, but resolves to try to spend more time in future with the staff involved with the patients he sees. He also makes himself available to talk things over with any staff who would like to see him, but the only member of staff who approaches him on this basis in the next few months is suicidal and needs to go off sick. He starts a research project on staff stress, with a view to presenting the results to the General Manager at the earliest opportunity. But overall he feels dissatisfied with his contribution as a consultant.

Comment

The psychiatrist felt unnecessarily overwhelmed. The modified approach to clinical referrals, involving more liaison and consultation with ward staff, was quite a good idea, and the research could be useful if it asked the right questions and was eventually presented in the right way. However, the open invitation to staff to approach him on demand was unlikely to be very productive, albeit his discovery of a suicidal student nurse.

On the other hand, he rightly perceived that any idea of the ward staff making regular use of an orderly, organised consultative group in the present situation was unrealistic. Given the duty rotas, it would be surprising if many nurses would be able to attend more than two or three meetings during the course of an attachment to the ward.

He might have found, however, that an offer to the medical, nursing, physiotherapy and occupational therapy staff to take a short series of seminars on such topics as facing death, giving bad news to patients, dealing with relatives' distress and managing personal stress would have been well received. Organising the seminars around case presentations, encouraging multi-disciplinary participation, and giving equal weight both to exploring feelings and practical management, would help make the subjects more real and alive. It would also help those considering making changes in how they worked to do so. The timing should be that which allowed the greatest number with the most information to attend; since this would be a consultative exercise, not a didactic one, these were the nurses.

Notes

(i)   The example and commentary illustrate what is in a way an ethical dilemma in consultative work. The consultant, in concluding that he could do nothing very much in response to the request, but undertook to put together systematic observations to present to the managers, was perhaps doing the right thing. He felt he was going to challenge the present working system in an orderly way, rather than risk shoring it up. On the other hand, research reports are commonly ignored.

(ii) The suggestion made in the commentary illustrates another strategy: modifying the consultative approach in the interests of the people who might benefit, yet without completely undermining its special qualities. The consultative seminar proposed in fact meets one of the key criteria of consultation – namely, to start where the other people were, and provide something not only useful but usable.

Example (3) continued: further developments

One of the nursing staff presents a case that is troubling her. An elderly woman, with what seems likely to be a terminal bout of a recurrent illness, has been expressing her extreme distress to her. She has been confiding in the nurse a complicated, somewhat bizarre and worrying story concerning her late husband and which could involve her daughter and son-in-law. It is an issue that is going to 'come out' sooner rather than later, especially if she should die, and could 'wreck her daughter's marriage'. The woman is fearful and depressed and tells the nurse that sometimes she just can't face the illness and her domestic worries and responsibilities, and she would rather 'end it all' now.

The nurse appears to give the patient more time than seems feasible. It emerges, to the nurse's own surprise, how much extra time for this patient she has been able to squeeze out of the day, at the expense of other duties. She has also started to pop into the ward when off duty, for a talk and also to run the occasional errand.

Is it realistic to do all this? Perhaps the task of helping this woman could be shared? The nurse says that she is the only person in whom the patient can confide. The patient says she can't talk to any of the other staff, and there seems to be mutual dislike with some. She says she cannot talk even to her daughter, who 'is going to have a shock when I die'; something to do with her background and a will.

During the consultation it is clear how distressed the nurse is about what she has taken on. She has never got to know someone so closely who is facing death. She wants to help but finds that all that happens is that she takes home each day a great weight of worries and sadness, only to be loaded with more the next day. She fears finding her dead one morning, and is losing sleep.

The ward sister, present in the meeting, is also unsure how to help, although she hadn't known how much time the nurse was spending with the patient, nor the alarm it was causing her. Why hadn't she discussed it with her?

Because the woman had asked her not to, and in fact had made her promise not to tell anyone about some other 'secrets', there was no way of discussing the woman's worries without revealing these, so the nurse felt trapped.

The discussion moves around to moving the nurse to another ward, or even moving the patient. The consultant asks the ward sister what she makes of the patient, and she reveals that what is happening is not so very different from what happened on her previous admission. Last time the ward sister suggested that the woman should see a social worker, but she wouldn't. She suspects she isn't telling the truth about her home life. She thinks she's mad.

The consultant points out that the nurse is not only trying to be a social worker and counsellor to the patient, but is being pulled into being a personal friend as well, almost like a relative. The nurse explains that her own mother was once very ill and she feared she was going to die, and this reminds her a little of that time. The consultant says that such experiences can make us more sensitive and less objective when something similar recurs in our work. It makes it even more important to be clear about professional roles.

How much flexibility is there for a nurse to spend more time with one patient than another? The ward sister confirms that there is very little time or flexibility, but if a nurse spends a few minutes more with one patient than another that's acceptable. But coming in off duty and running errands isn't. As a general rule, or in this particular case? The ward sister considers; then makes it clear, speaking directly to the nurse, that in this particular woman's case it is inadvisable.

It is agreed that the nurse should not distance herself from the woman. The option to sanction the amount of time the nurse spends with the woman, but with supervision of the work, is decided to be impracticable. The ward sister and nurse suggest that instead the woman should see a social worker about her domestic problem.

'Or a lawyer?' asks the consultant. It shouldn't be assumed that only a hospital worker can help. Why not leave it to the woman to decide? There are also her feelings about her illness and impending death. Could she see the chaplain, or the psychiatrist, if she wished?

The turn of the discussion is making the nurse uneasy. They discuss death, and the group concludes that impending death makes someone seem special, and the usual professional approaches don't seem easy to apply. They go on to discover that it is the absence of formal permission, methods, training or even discussion about facing death that can lead to individual members of staff feeling guilty and helpless and going their own way, which is what the nurse did.

In the event, ward sister and nurse see the woman together for twenty useful minutes which produce tears and relief, and the woman decides that there is something for her lawyer and for the social worker to help her with. The limited time the nurse and the patient spend together now appears more helpful to the woman, and just before her death she thanks the nurse for her kindness.

Notes

(i) The consultation has followed a difficult path between the nurse's personal feelings and background on the one hand and on the other the ward's (indeed the hospital's) lack of a policy for dealing with feelings. However, taking this in-between course has involved touching on these two areas rather than ignoring them, and it is possible that the nurse will have learned something professionally helpful for herself, and the ward sister something equally useful for the way she runs her team.

(ii) The consultant was intrigued by the woman's story. From the nurse's account both the woman's personality and mental state, and her family situation, seemed to have areas worth pursuing; indeed at one point he wondered whether she was more ill than she seemed, and that the mysterious family story was delusional. But he was undertaking consultation with the nurse, not supervising a clinical case, and concluded on balance that what they were dealing with was a very sad and rather muddled lady with some family problems, perhaps amplified by her circumstances. Was it just possible that the patient had a major treatable mental illness, a severe personality disorder that could cause someone serious trouble, or even a brain tumour? Yes.

(iii) The junior nurse wasn't unusually mature or sensible, and the ward sister not outstanding. Both, however, were competent people doing their best in difficult circumstances, and it was correct for the consultant to respect their respective positions and guide the meeting so that, at one point, the ward sister in effect demonstrated her supervisory role within the consultation. The other disciplines present, although contributing ideas, were not encouraged to make this a multidisciplinary matter, which was not the way the ward worked. Had someone thought of it, a physiotherapist or occupational therapist could have suggested how their respective work might have contributed. The consultant was unsure about the junior doctor's position, and how far the issue was a nursing or medical one. However, the patient's own house physician participated in the consultation and was aware of the issues, and that was left at that.

(iv) In all quite a lot was achieved, educationally as well as for the nurse and the woman, by a forty-five minute consultation followed by the twenty minute session the two nurses had with the patient. A great deal of unproductive and even damaging time and effort was saved.

(v) This example has portrayed a stereotypical theme which is frequently aired. On the one hand there is the essentially autocratically-led general hospital, where the ethos is to get on with the job without the distracting or even undermining effect of getting involved with patients and their feelings. Feelings are not ignored, but are handled on a brisk, friendly, no-nonsense, stiff-upper-lip basis, with jokes, reassurance and encouragement freely ladled out, and a certain amount of contempt in reserve for the more feeble members of the community – patients or staff. For the really awkward or miserable, the psychiatrist may be summoned, it being felt that they deserve each other.

On the other hand there is the psychiatrist or the social worker, afloat like the chaplain on a slightly different plane, wise, understanding, sharing, caring and so forth, tolerated for a time while the preliminaries for decisions are gone through.

These are caricatures, but not so very far from the pictures often held on each side. Probably most readers of this book would agree that compassion and the exploration of feelings on the part of the social worker, or psychiatrist, or chaplain is not to be despised; but up to a point a certain amount of firmness and briskness and the containment of feelings is not to be automatically dismissed or despised either, providing it coexists with courtesy, humanity and technical competence. Once more, it is a question of balance, and to help find the point of balance between how the organisation works and how the consultant feels it should work, he or she should not jump to premature conclusions, but begin by trying to see the job through the eyes of the consultees.

(4) An in-patient psychiatric unit

The consultant directing an in-patient unit asked the hospital's Anglican chaplain, who is trained in consultation and group work, to take a weekly staff group. The group is still going after fourteen years, with consultant and consultees continuing to learn about it.

At the outset no clear rules or contract were defined, although in a paper summarising his experience the group's consultant recommends a clear, written contract for the staff and the group's leader (Foskett, 1986).

The group meets weekly, and senior staff (consultant psychiatrist, senior charge nurse, senior social workers, occupational therapist) are usually present, plus the junior medical staff, who are expected to attend. In other respects attendance varies considerably, usually about fifteen or twenty people in all but occasionally more. This represents about two-thirds of the people on the unit at the time, non-attenders including some teachers who have chosen not to attend, plus teachers and nurses supervising patients. Several part-time staff don't have the staff group in their timetable.

The work of the group is almost always to do with current feelings and working relationships. A meeting will characteristically begin with a range of comments about the group (about being late, about who's there or not there) and then lapses into silence. The group is used to twenty minute silences, sometimes tense, sometimes to do with waiting for the right topic to emerge, occasionally calm and even restful.

Certain processes recur. For example, a member of staff will express strong feelings: irritation, distress, anger, or feelings of helplessness. Others will respond with rational explanations and advice. The group's consultant points out the difference. Different participants point out the respective pros and cons of being rational and objective. Someone then gets very angry.

The shifting discussion and feelings are always about a current theme on the unit: a painful event in the last few days, pressures of work from within or without, people leaving and joining the staff, feelings of anxiety, anger or helplessness about one or other patient, anger between staff members about something done or not done, said or not said. The participants vary, though with a regular, mostly senior core; there is always a sense of intensity, and often enough a sense of some work done and also of work not done. The meeting ends precisely on time. No decisions are made, but strong views are expressed, forged or clarified, and characteristically emerge in a week or two at one of the policy-making meetings, as a proposal. Once or twice a year the proposal is to hold an all-day meeting to explore something more fully. These meetings are planned in detail by a small working party, and may be experiential, administrative or both.

Comment

The meeting's main problem is in involving a sufficient proportion of the staff. With the exception of two or three conscientious objectors, most non-attenders have commitments either to a duty rota or two other branches of the organisation, miles away, which could only be challenged by a determined inquisition. It was decided not to do this.

Instead, there is an expectation that people will attend, and this is reinforced from time to time. But in general the group's viability is in its persistence; it rolls on and on over the years with the same facilitator and myself, promptly at the same time and place each week. This is one strength, the other being the skills, strength and persistence of the group's outside consultant.

The group has difficulty with dealing with feelings alone; that is to say, after a little time they tend to be diverted in some way, often into activity or rational conversation. This is the hospital's style, and is also a function of the high rate of staff in training passing through; which again is a characteristic of the hospital. On the more positive side, the participants seem often to be struggling with how best to manage and express real feelings in a way that is useful to the group, and while people often divert in one or another, it is rarely into jargon, interpretation or psychological clichés.

Notes

(i)   Is it a consultative group? It meets the criteria given in Chapter 1, its starting point being how the staff, not the consultant, perceive their work and methods and it operates at a social dynamic level, which corresponds with the working style of the unit.

(ii)   The group was an experiment which has grown and developed its own rules and procedures, most of which are referred to or implied above. It is a model that would fit some psychiatric units' needs, but for others, particularly where the emphasis of treatment and teaching was primarily psychodynamic or sociodynamic, tighter controls of participation would probably be advisable.

(iii) In many ways the meeting operates as a team and unit development group (see Chapter 6) despite its changing membership. It is rarely client-centred, although issues to do with patients are commonly the stimulus for the group's work on mutual feelings and relationships. To this extent it tends to operate somewhere between client and group foci in the short-term, with organisation development as the longer-term goal.

Chapter 5

Consultation in Practice II: Examples in Different Circumstances

Introduction

Interprofessional consultation must be adaptable to an extraordinarily wide range of quite different needs and situations. In this chapter examples will be given of:

(1) consultation in a crisis;
(2) consultation adapted to the case conference;
(3) a consultative-diagnostic strategy;
(4) a consultative group for student counsellors.

(1) Consultation in a crisis

Here are two examples:

• A telephone call to a psychiatric unit describes a young man with a history of depression who has now become increasingly excited and elated over the past few days. This is despite increasing doses of medication which are failing to sedate him, while possibly adding to his confusion. He is awake and noisy all night, and behaving in a bizarre and chaotic way by day, including hurrying up and down the street engaging the neighbours in conversations which lead rapidly to mounting irritation on one side or the other. There has already been some damage done, and today there was quite a serious fight. He hasn't been eating for some days, and has now stopped drinking. He keeps changing his mind about whether or not to accept admission to hospital. His wife is asking for something to be done urgently.

After a short telephone discussion arrangements are made to see the patient immediately as an emergency, with a view to direct admission to hospital, compulsorily if necessary.

• A telephone call to a psychiatric unit describes a young man in his late teens who this evening has got into a drunken fight with his father, was subsequently thrown out of the house, broke some windows and is now in the local police station. There have been similar events before. He is described as being full of remorse and depressed. He has been depressed in the past, and treated by his family doctor with antidepressants. He wants to go home but his father is still angry with him. The police are planning to charge him and detain him for his own safety unless a place can be found at once in a psychiatric hospital. The caller is the family doctor; the boy's mother, distraught at the prospects of either further trouble at home or a night in the cells for her son, is pleading with the general practitioner to do something.

What are the issues? In the second example, the family doctor has been landed with a difficult situation: his patient's mother is in the surgery pleading for action; the young man, mental state unknown, is in the police station where he may stay the night; home and father are somewhere else.

On the one hand the patient may be depressed, and in the past has even ruminated about suicide. On the other he was never seriously mentally ill, has kept a job and a girl friend, and the present crisis sounds more like a domestic dispute, albeit a serious one, than a situation demanding the young man's emergency admission to hospital.

The pressure for action is coming from the young man's mother. But information is lacking and a great deal unknown, and it cannot be simply assumed that the young man isn't fit to go home, or that a renewed fight will break out if he does. The young man's mother may be right, that the situation at home is in one way or the other untenable, or in her distress she may be more fearful than is justified. One way of getting all the information needed (about the patient's state, and about the likely outcome of whichever option is chosen) would be to arrange a family meeting at the police station. The family doctor thinks this impracticable, and he is too busy now to go and see the patient himself.

The GP, clear that the required step at this stage is information gathering rather than action, suggests that the police call their police surgeon to assess whether the patient is severely depressed or even suicidal, because this is the clinical decision on which possible next steps will depend.

If he isn't, the immediate matter is a legal and social one. The health visitor isn't available, and the experience of both the general practitioner and the psychiatrist is that the social services department is too overstretched to deal with this case on an emergency basis, although they should still be approached if all else fails.

The GP decides to tell the mother that whatever the outcome of this evening's crisis, the longer term situation must somehow be resolved at home if their son is to live there. They can either leave things as they are and live with the consequences, make a decision as a family to deal with the father-son dispute and the son's heavy drinking, or require him to leave home. It is up to her and her husband to decide, with or without outside help, e.g. from the Social Services Department or citizen's advice bureau.

The GP says he will speak to the young man's mother along these lines, and will suggest that she and her husband go along to the police station while he phones them about involving the police surgeon, whom he knows.

Later he phones back to say that the police say the young man has sobered up, has had a meal and would like to patch things up with his father, and suggests staying with his aunt for the weekend. His mother confirms that they get on well, that this is a good idea, and that father and son have shaken hands and agreed that they must sort things out next week. They decide not to call in the police surgeon after all.

In due course the young man is fined in court, and the GP arranges a family appointment with a social worker. They do not keep it.

Notes

(i)   This second example is a classically messy situation involving multiple people and agencies, which might once have been resolved either by a night in the cells or by a short and unsatisfactory admission to a psychiatric unit.

In the telephoned consultation the issues explored were essentially whether the hospital unit had what the young man needed. It seemed that the most important and immediate need was for breathing space while tempers cooled, and the longer term need was for something to be done to help the young man live with his family or leave. If the latter practical issue were explored properly, it would also throw light on whether individual psychiatric or psychological help had a place.

The outcome was likely to be more helpful to the young man than hospital admission; at the same time the consultation served to divert, correctly, a domestic and legal situation away from a psychiatric solution, which if not actually imposed was nearly seized upon in the heat of the crisis. The possibility of choosing psychiatric help in due course, with adequate time for a thorough assessment of how much it would help, of course remained open.

(ii)   In the first example consultation was potential rather than actual, because the first few moments of discussion clearly described a person whose problems were likely to need, as urgently as possible, clinical assessment, treatment and observation by a medical and nursing team around the clock.

(2) Consultation adapted to the case conference

Case conferences are by no means necessarily consultative. Some are occasions when information is shared so that different people involved in a case know what each other are doing. Others involve different participants, perhaps of different disciplines, contributing information and views to a clinical or otherwise case-centred plan of action. This might be one person's decision (e.g. a medical consultant or senior social worker) or the conference may reach its conclusions by consensus.

A case conference is consultative when it represents two or more groups or agencies, and begins without any assumptions about which will in the end be responsible for what: the purpose of the consultation is to see what is needed and who is in the best position to provide it.

For example, a psychiatrist at one children's hospital refers an anorexic teenager to another psychiatric in-patient unit. He feels he has made no progress with the girl, and indeed she was previously in another unit which also passed her on after failing to help. Moreover, her parents are distressed and complaining and demanding further opinions.

The psychiatrist's expectation is that the girl and her family will be offered an appointment for a clinical assessment, with a view to the next psychiatric team taking over.

Instead, the second child psychiatrist suggests coming with a colleague (a nurse) to join in the next routine case conference that they hold. At this meeting the team currently looking after the girl present the history in detail, and review their attempts at treatment. This includes many failed attempts to involve the girl's family in work. The pattern that emerges is of initial success and weight gain until discharge is planned with lengthening periods at home, at which point she becomes more difficult to treat and loses weight. The parents, both busy professional people, with the father often out of the country, expressed a willingness to take part in family therapy, but sessions tend to end in arguments about their not knowing what the sessions are for, with the therapist asking them what *they* think.

This leads to a discussion about styles of family therapy, how much to meet the parents half-way with the logical explanations they want, how much to face them with less commonsensical responses. The first unit's achievements are noted, and also the areas where they have come unstuck.

The second unit now offers the family (all of them) an appointment. There is no need to spend time taking a detailed history and repeating the individual psychiatric assessment; this has already been competently done. Instead the meeting is more like a crisis meeting, putting the questions: where do we go from here, who is going to undertake to do what, and what part will the parents play? If the girl loses weight when discharge is planned, then they have two things to consider. Perhaps returning home isn't in fact wanted, and alternatives should be considered? Or might it be that if the parents were involved in mealtimes from the start, feeding problems at home would be tackled and helped throughout, rather than emerging again when the nurses were, so to speak, handing her back?

Notes

(i)   The notion of a fresh start with a second team making a thorough reassessment was tempting to all concerned, and at times is appropriate. But the first team had the benefit of a vast amount of information about problems, management and progress and the benefit of this was gained in the way described.

(ii) This also freed the first meeting with the second team to go straight to the point: not only that progress needed to be made and sustained, but that there was concern to explore every avenue to prevent a third failure. So what had they all (family and clinicians) learned from what had happened so far? It did seem that one thing to be avoided was the psychiatric team doing something for the girl that couldn't be sustained at home. What is important here is not the change of strategy, but that the consultative meeting enabled the second unit to get off to a more effective fresh start.

(iii) The consultative meeting need not necessarily have resulted in the transfer of the patient's care. This was a matter for both the teams, the girl and her family. The consultation could have resulted in the first unit carrying on, in the light of the review of progress held with the help of outside peers, and with a modified approach to the work with the parents.

(3) A consultative-diagnostic strategy

A probation officer is working with a young man with a profoundly disturbed personality. She is the first professional worker to forge a useful working relationship with him. Over the longer period he is making real progress; but every so often he becomes profoundly depressed and for a few days becomes self-destructive, causing anxiety in the probation hostel where he lives, and threatening to injure himself. The staff there feel he is more than they can handle at such times, and that he ought to be treated in hospital. They feel he is really quite ill when depressed.

In consultation with a psychiatrist the probation officer describes his long history of very disturbed relationships. In childhood there were several changes of children's home. His recurrent spells of depression seem understandable in the light of this. The following emerge from the consultation:

(a) The probation officer is satisfied that she is making real progress; she and the client feel so, and the facts of the past year (offences practically ended, though replaced by spells of sadness) support this. Nevertheless, the emotional problems that have emerged are serious.
(b) The hostel is a good one, and takes a broadly therapeutic approach. The probation officer is anxious not to lose the place her client has there, but the staff are anxious, uncharacteristically so, and his place is undoubtedly threatened.
(c) The psychiatrist isn't sure whether or not the client's depression is entirely psychosocial in origin. There might be a place for medication; there are questions she would like to ask about his symptoms and family background, if it can be traced.

The psychiatrist and probation officer agree that the psychiatrist should see her client, of course with his agreement and that of the hostel's general practitioner. Psychiatrist and probation officer meet the hostel staff, and the impression is of an experienced team who know that they are managing confidently and well until the occasional few days of despair and agitation that overcome the client from time to time.

Having met the client and the hostel staff, the psychiatrist offers to see the man at very short notice, with a view to an immediate but brief crisis admission, whenever a similar depressive episode occurs.

This offer appears to relieve the situation. It is taken up once a few weeks later, and doesn't seem needed again. From the psychiatrist's contact with the probation officer's client, she concludes that medication isn't indicated.

Notes

(i) The work of both probation officer and the hostel, and an unusual period of continuity in the man's life, have been preserved. The price of doing so has been sufficient psychiatric intervention to confirm that a full transfer to psychiatric care is not necessary, and indeed is contra-indicated.

(ii) The value of taking both a consultative and a 'medical model' approach is clearer if their differences are understood (Steinberg, 1983; Tyrer and Steinberg, 1987).

As stated earlier, the bedrock of the medical approach is not the assumption of physical causes and treatments, but diagnosis of the other person's state of disorder, according to the diagnostician's conceptual models and what he believes he perceives in what the other person says and does.

The consultative approach is quite distinct. As has been pointed out, the consultative approach uses the consultee's way of seeing things and the consultee's methods and skills.

If the differences are clear, then both approaches can be used in a particular person's interests without jeopardising the value of either, and without blurring the boundaries of the different professionals' roles and responsibilities. In this example, the psychiatrist so to speak 'had a look' at the client, and then withdrew, having satisfied herself that affirming the availability of her psychiatric service if necessary was on balance more likely to maintain the client with his existing helpers than if she had remained completely uninvolved.

It might have been that the man's mental state would have justified a trial period on an antidepressant drug, or a mood-stabiliser like lithium. Again, the psychiatrist could have contributed this aspect of care, while the probation officer and the hostel staff continued with theirs, with continuing consultation used to ensure that the contributions from different people were still useful, and properly co-ordinated. It is a very useful approach in work which is likely to involve several agencies, for example in clinical work with young people (Steinberg, 1986a, 1987).

(4) A consultative group for student counsellors

A group of counsellors from colleges of further education meet a psychologist regularly throughout term time. Some of them have supervision provided in their own work settings, one or two meet colleagues to discuss cases, most have no such provision at all. They meet at a centre away from their places of work, and with the permission of whoever are their seniors. One counsellor finds even this preliminary aspect of consultation illuminating: she finds that there is no-one in the college to whom she is responsible. It seems that the right person, technically, is the vice-principal. This comes as something of a revelation to him, but he is pleased to hear that she exists, and about her work.

In the consultative meetings the counsellors share ideas and feelings with people they do not ordinarily meet in their work, and look at their clients' cases from this new perspective. On each occasion, a counsellor presents a piece of his or her current work, either because it is of interest or because there is a problem. The work they are doing is primarily with individual students, and concerns emotional, relationship, family, academic and career problems. Occasionally something more pressing emerges, e.g. an unwanted pregnancy, drug misuse or a clash with the law.

The meetings are run as consultative seminars, that is to say consultants and consultees are aware of the educational as well as problem-solving value of the sessions, and occasionally a consultant or consultee proposes a general topic for a meeting, for example to share ideas and information about drug abuse or AIDS, or suggests using a technique like sculpting, role play or videotape. From the start the meetings have a built-in life span of a year overall, during which time they are not open to new participants. At the end of each term a meeting is set aside to review progress, and an attempt made to record and evaluate the group's progress and achievements.

Notes

(i)   The work is essentially client-centred, but there are fre-
      quent shifts of focus to the consultees' work, individually or
      as a group. In a study of a similar group (mentioned earlier)
      Steinberg and Hughes (1987) noticed a tendency as consul-
      tative groups became established for the consultees to seem
      to find less need to bring their clients' cases to the meetings,
      and instead to raise work issues to do with their roles,
      supervision etc. These areas of difficulty often seemed a
      greater challenge to their work than were their clients'
      problems.

(ii) Planning a regular consultative group of this sort requires
      the same careful thought as holding a regular group in an
      institution. Decisions need to be made at the start about
      permission to participate, membership, frequency of meet-
      ing and how and when the series of meetings will end, and
      about any built-in evaluation.

(iii) However sophisticated the consultees, clarification of the
      purpose of the group is always important.

(iv) Confidentiality issues can be particularly prominent in a
      group of this sort. This is discussed in Chapter 7.

Chapter 6

Consultation in Practice III: Staff, Team and Group Development

Introduction

We have seen that interprofessional consultation may be primarily problem-orientated, with new learning and professional development as a by-product; or vice-versa, with training and development as the main aim.

In training and development programmes the stimulus and focus for the consultative work is the goal identified by the consultees; it does not have to be a 'problem'. (It can be unhelpful that problems tend to be perceived as inherently 'bad', i.e. they represent failure and should be avoidable and are a cause for embarrassment, while personal or organisational development is seen as 'good'. Ideally it is all relative; consultation should help people get from A to B whatever the reason for change.)

In this chapter examples will be given of:

(1) training consultation: individual psychotherapy consultation to an adolescent unit;
(2) consulting to a service in a different culture;
(3) a service development programme;
(4) a teaching workshop taken on consultative lines.

(1) Individual psychotherapy consultation to an adolescent unit

A psychiatric unit working with adolescent in-patients asks a senior psychotherapist to take a regular consultative group, with the dynamics of dyadic staff-patient relationships as the focus. There is a great variety of paired relationships: there may be psychotherapy, art therapy, dramatherapy, occupational therapy or counselling as part of the prescribed treatment programmes; but the boys and girls spend time with staff for other reasons ('seeing the doctor', being taught in class, living in the ward and so on) as well as developing friendly relationships of varying degrees of intensity with staff they select themselves.

The cases and situations presented to the consultant in succeeding weeks include, for example: an impasse in psychotherapy, discussed in the group with both therapist and supervisor; the question of how much in a psychotherapy session should remain private within the therapeutic relationship, and how much shared; the suitability or otherwise of a particular patient for psychotherapy, and which type; a patient who is not using counselling sessions but is talking extensively to another member of staff; a patient who is confiding in a number of different people; a nurse who is finding a relationship with one of the patients difficult – she attends the group with her own nursing supervisor.

Each consultation is about a patient's case, or about a situation, and not about an abstract topic. Each meeting ends with the various points ventilated and examined rather than necessarily cleared up, and the consultation is complete in itself, with no planned continuity, although the same case may be presented again another time.

Notes

(i)   The meeting has characteristics of a seminar, but one which is focussed around a particular case and a particular question – something in the area of the psychodynamics of pair-relationships with which the presenter or the team want help and clarification. It is in this sense that this type of teaching is consultative.

(ii)   The meeting doesn't provide supervision. With reference to Figure 1.2, a nurse presenting a case may, for example, also be having both (a) supervision of his psychotherapeutic work by a senior psychiatric registrar, and (b) supervision of his work as a nurse by the senior nurse on his ward.

(iii) The meeting is one from which participants may take new ideas, attitudes and feelings but not formal decisions. Plans are not made in this meeting but elsewhere.

It follows from (ii) and (iii) that the consultant is not responsible for that patient's management, nor does he propose that plans made in clinical management meetings should change; on the other hand he will make observations that may reveal discrepancies between the direction of thinking in the consultative group and decisions made elsewhere.

If the team or organisation and the consultant are clear about the respective functions of the consultative group and the clinical management meetings, then the consultative group can function unfettered as a highly valuable source of teaching and ideas, which of course may have impact on the decision-making meetings. But it does so by widening and deepening the experience of individuals who attend the management meeting. Its authority is therefore invested in its function as a forum for study and teaching, rather than as part of the managerial (clinical and administrative) structure.

If an organisation is not clear about the distinction between the functions of the consultative group and the managerial structure, or if the latter lacks strength or ideas of its own, then the enormous benefits of the consultative meetings are lost, and at worst the managerial structure may appear threatened.

These and related multidisciplinary issues are discussed in accounts of family therapy consultation (Dare, 1986) and individual psychotherapy consultation (Wilson, 1986) in an adolescent unit, and from the unit's perspective as a whole in Steinberg (1986a).

(2) Consulting to a service in a different culture

An experienced residential care worker is asked to provide consultation in a community very different from his own, perhaps in another country, about the development of a therapeutic hostel and services associated with it.

The invitation is accepted. Much of the preliminary work may be done by correspondence, despite which certain aspects of what is hoped for may remain unclear, and the consultant may not be sure how much is due to language differences (which there can be, even when the shared language is on the face of it the same, e.g. English) and how much is due to the careful mutual courtesies which go with this sort of invitation.

The consultant decides to postpone detailed discussion about what is expected of the consultation, and about working at the most effective level, until the consultation starts. In an attempt to make up for some of the uncertainty, he discusses with people who are apparently familiar with that culture or that community what they may be hoping for in the consultation, and what they have to work with (facilities, staffing, resources).

On arrival, he finds his schedule and the people participating already arranged in detail, partly and partly not in accordance with what was discussed in advance. He has a sense of politics and diplomacy being influential in the programme of consultation, the lists of participants and in any precedence he detects. He may also find himself unexpectedly asked to do something quite different as well, e.g. to deliver a lecture about a model therapeutic hostel. He has doubts about aspects of all this, but a sense of mutual carefulness and courtesy tends to inhibit questions and suggestions.

Notes

(i)   It isn't necessary to travel for example to Beijing to find a difference in background culture that immediately challenges the ground rules of consultation. A social worker among surgeons or a psychiatrist in a convent may discover an equally distinctively different ambience.

   The information sought in advance should be as much about the people and the culture or subculture from the widest point of view, and not only about the particular development that is the focus of consultation, nor only about the professions involved. Advice from individuals should be seen in perspective. It is likely to be the truth but not the whole truth, and the aspiring consultant, anxious and enthusiastic to develop a complete picture, may jump to unwarranted conclusions about the likely scene.

(ii) The subject for consultation may be too wide. As the short time available passes the consultant may not be sure which would concern him most – the recommendations that emerge being abandoned, or the whole lot being accepted uncritically and unchallenged as part of a five- or ten-year scheme. It is preferable to negotiate about different consultative meetings or study groups looking at aspects of the subject, e.g. sources of information about the existing state of affairs, how it has been evaluated, where requests for change are coming from, how much change is expected, training issues, and so on, rather than being tempted to deal with too universal an issue. However, if time is short the most useful consultation may be about precisely this, i.e. breaking large issues down into manageable size.

(iii) Language differences are not necessarily a problem. A careful, non-intrusive interpreter who shares the consultant's and the consultees' concern about dealing as precisely as possible with meanings and concepts, and a group that does not mind taking time to ensure that what is being said is fully understood, may add up to a more illuminating consultation than one where people only think they understand each other. It can be helpful if those who will interpret are some of the consultees. A preliminary consultation with them, to look at questions of communication, and to clarify the ground rules and requirements of consultation, can be extremely helpful. (This is an example of the role reversal which should come easily in consultation: the consultant-to-be consults with the consultees-to-be about how to operate most effectively for them.)

(iv) It is the culture difference, and the carefulness and tentativeness about discussion which can mark occasions when cultural differences are most felt, that can make difficult the frank, probing questioning and clarifying which is fundamental to consultation. This fact, if it happens to be the case, should itself be a preliminary focus for acknowledgement and discussion. The consultant should not be afraid to be naive and curious, because asking simple questions and if necessary lots of them is the basis of the art.

(3) A service development programme

Consultation is sought by a large welfare organisation which wants to shift the emphasis of its work from a residential to a community-based service. The consultative task is to look at the organisation's training needs, and the consultant is asked to work with a group which has already been set up with this task in mind.

The organisation has already worked out the broad changes which will happen in terms of buildings and staffing and timescale. The consultant is told about this at an early stage, and smartly suited people with organiser files and briefcases, using the latest management jargon, provide him with volumes of beautifully bound and printed management plans and flow sheets.

Everything seems most thoroughly thought out, everything having been thought of from epidemiology and the wishes of the client group to the detailed cash flows involved. The organisation's management makes it clear that the specific task for the consultant is to do with training; what type of training, carried out by whom, retraining of existing staff where necessary, recruitment and induction of new staff and so on.

The consultant's own feeling is that things are so highly organised and clear-cut that if it doesn't work perfectly it may not work at all. He feels uneasy from the outset, because he is more comfortable working with group feelings, while the consultees seem more oriented to working intellectually and on paper. He does not feel it would be right to step in too soon with a direct criticism based on his own assumptions, and 'consults with himself' about how his misgivings may matter.

It seems that there is a flaw in the plans. Consultation will of course have no point if it is assumed from the start that the consultative process will not generate new thinking in the consultees; yet everything is so tightly planned that the various schedules do not seem flexible enough to accommodate anything new that emerges. The consultant has some further ideas around this theme but does not want to think it through too far ahead without the consultees. He suggests that they make time for a longer session, a half-day or if possible a whole day, mid-week or weekend as they wish, to look at the issue of *adaptability* during the year or two of consultation leading to institutional change.

The suggestion, which the consultant framed with various alternatives in order to be helpful, throws the group into disarray. They are suddenly unsure about the value of such a meeting, a little anxious about what form it will take, unclear how they will decide among themselves whether and when to have it, and not certain whether they can make this decision or should refer it back to higher management. The group seems quite disabled and a little depressed. The consultant leads them round to thinking about how they ordinarily solve problems, and they decide that they would prefer to elect a chairman and go through somewhat more formal procedures to make the necessary decisions and get the necessary permissions for the longer meeting. It is certainly clear that without these permissions the consultant will by no means be sure of getting a fee for the longer meeting.

In the event a whole day session is planned, with small group and large group meetings around the theme of the organisation's likely training needs. The consultant resists the idea of a formal agenda, but encourages the idea that the consultees will record on flip-charts the sort of ideas that come up, and at the end of the day will get together on a slightly more formal basis to draw up their conclusions in a form they feel the organisation can use.

The consultant suggests a simple exercise. The group divides into three. One group spends some time planning a model training scheme for helping staff cope with difficult clients in the home. Another group plans a day attendance centre's daily programme. The two groups then get together with the third, whose task is to integrate the training scheme with the day centre's programme. They are surprised how difficult the latter task is, and find that training needs and service needs seem inseparable. The day began as one which the consultees resisted, and then tolerated. It ends, however, not only with a new discovery about the likely interdependence of training and service needs in their development plans, but also the experience that this new learning of their own required changing some of their own assumptions and methods, and not without a little discomfort. They decide to build into their plans machinery for evaluating and if necessary modifying developments.

Notes

(i) The consultant held a fine balance between stating very directly what he thought was amiss with the organisation's methods, and helping them find out for themselves. By holding back from giving a diagnosis and making prescriptions he enabled the consultees to find something out for themselves and gave them the opportunity of becoming more innovative and adaptable in the process.

(ii) Another balance sought by the consultant was between using approaches he thought appropriate for the task, for example introducing a much longer session and using experiential exercises, and the use of the consultees' own methods, e.g. the committee meeting to resolve an early problem. The consultant correctly starts with the consultees' approaches, but introduces new ideas for them to try.

(iii) Similarly, it was helpful for the consultative group to explore the uses, for different purposes, of the consultees' highly organised, cognitive style and the experiential approach the consultant wanted to introduce. The consultant should have a range of consultative 'tools' in his bag to offer the consultees for their work, as well as being open to their suggestions. This often amounts to something of a personal struggle for the consultant, who will often think he or she knows best, while being conscious of the opposing requirement to help the consultees set their own tasks and use their own methods. Again, it should not be a matter of either the consultant or the consultees getting their own way, but of setting the balance in the right place, and by mutual agreement.

(iv) The consultation demonstrated the common and useful phenomenon of changes occurring at more than one level; in the consultative group itself, in the organisation, and at the level of personal learning. Thus the move from being stuck with the original plan to introducing the longer session, and then the eventual successful use of that session:

(a) involved work and achievement in reorganising the programme itself;

(b) demonstrated something worth knowing about the wider organisation and the possible conflict that could arise between its aims and its methods;

(c) served as a model through which the consultees discovered that an approach they had neither foreseen nor allowed for turned out to advance their thinking, experience and information.

(4) A teaching workshop taken on consultative lines

The task is to use art techniques to explore the theme of creativity and its constraints in psychiatry. The point in question is made as clear as possible in the introduction to the workshop, and explained in a brief written handout: that therapists need to be creative in developing and carrying out treatments, that patients need to be creative in making use of therapy, coping with problems and accomplishing change, and that organising and improving therapeutic services requires creative thinking and activity too. But there are constraints in psychiatric and therapeutic practice: issues of risk and safety, ethical questions, the limitations inherent in psychiatric disorders, the institutional limits set by the organisation, and the cultural, social and legal constraints set by the wider community, all this quite apart from the limits to our understanding of psychiatric conditions and their treatment.

The person leading the workshop is a psychiatrist who uses art techniques in teaching and treatment. The participants are course members and their teachers at an arts and therapy centre. They are from various backgrounds, for example psychology, social work and occupational therapy, and are engaged in training to use creative techniques such as art and drama in their therapeutic work. The aim is to study and learn about the topic. The process is consultative because at the outset the teacher has no idea what will emerge. He has made clear his own reasons for thinking that the subject is important, and it is understood that his primary task is to help the class explore it, but he also assumes that by the end of the two days he will have learned at least as much as the participants. The workshop is held abroad, in a foreign language, the senior staff participants acting as interpreters.

The workshop begins with a large group discussion around the general themes of creativity, the psychotherapies, psychiatry, the participants' own professions and experience, and the constraints they experience. These include personal anxieties and difficulties in undertaking work with patients,

patients' problems, and all sorts of institutional problems. Conceptual and philosophical problems, limitations on our knowledge and problems in extending it are discussed. To keep the ideas literally in sight words, phrases and the odd sketch and doodle from this 'brainstorming' session are written up on a sheet occupying half the wall, which is soon filled.

This is followed by an exercise in small groups: each participant produces a picture representing an aspect of his or her work. The groups then see what the pictures and the process of producing them illustrate about work and personal creativity. Themes that emerge are to do with anxiety and inhibitions, assertiveness, the taking of risks, personal exposure, getting stuck, knowing but not being able to explain, making assumptions which turn out to be wrong, and so on. These are discussed in the larger group in relation to one's work. Later there is a related exercise in which groups of five or six people produce group paintings, exploring creativity, risks, and constraints in cooperative work. The advantages and problems of collaborative work are explored: euphoria and gloom, enjoyment and anger, opportunity and limitations are experienced.

The consultant, himself intermittently consulting with the course teachers, comments on developments in the group dynamics as the day proceeds. The final session is spent reviewing the day and what was learned, 'fixing' some of the experiences, observations and feelings in words, and helping the group 'back to earth'. The second day is similar in form and on the theme of working with constraints in a positive way.

Notes

(i)   The example is of consultation with teaching as the primary aim. Its particularly consultative characteristic lies in the principal role undertaken by the consultant, which is to encourage and guide a learning occasion rather than to convey information. In this example several participants had more experience than the consultant in the practice of creative therapies, for example.

(ii) For these reasons the occasion was to a considerable extent a peer exercise in joint learning: the consultant, although with ideas of his own about the subject, could not know what would be learned from the workshop.

(iii) It is also a characteristic of consultation that the process includes generating new ideas and the making of new observations, and a wider study of the subject than would be required only for personal learning or problem-solving. It is more like a form of study than a way of imparting technical expertise.

(iv) In the move along the consultative spectrum from crisis intervention and problem-solving to consultation as a teaching method, the notion of the core work problem changes. In some examples the problem is an immediate one, for example how to handle a clinical situation that seems unmanageable. In other examples the problem is more to do with something amiss in the management process itself. When the emphasis is on new learning and new developments, the challenge is no less real, but it does tend to be seen in a different light, and appear less climactic than it is.

Chapter 7

Problems, Ethics and Evaluation in Consultative Work

Some problems

Problems and pitfalls of consultation that have already been mentioned include:

(1) 'mandated' consultation
(2) going in at the wrong level;
(3) misunderstandings about what consultation entails;
(4) misunderstandings about the consultee's autonomy and role;
(5) drifting into clinical work;
(6) slipping into psychotherapy
(7) sliding into politics and administration;
(8) being too rigid about the 'rules' given in Chapter 3.

Mandated consultation, to use Caplan's term (1970), where A proposes that B 'needs' consultation, is only a problem if points 2, 3 and 4 are handled without care. It is essential that the consultee has an aim for consultation, and that the consultee's work and responsibility look broadly co-extensive with the likely focus and range of the consultation. Suppose a Director of Social Services asked a consultant to provide consultation to a group of children's homes because the milieux there were insufficiently psychotherapeutic. The consultant would need to clarify whether this was a departmental policy decision which had been agreed with all concerned, including the children's home staff, or whether the children's homes wished to develop their work in this direction, and had permission to do so; and that it was at least feasible that staffing and training resources could be reviewed in the light of what emerged. If the consultant were to 'go in' without knowing the answers to these questions there would be the risk of a great deal of discomfort and wasted time.

Moving from consultation into *clinical or psychotherapeutic work*, or getting involved in *policy discussions*, is a matter of fine judgement. A consultant may seem rigid and unhelpful if he too assiduously avoids these high risk areas, just as the work could become something other than consultation if he crosses these boundaries without caution. To take one example, if a psychiatrist or psychologist were undertaking client-centred consultation at a school or children's home it would be reasonable not to rule out occasionally seeing children there. But it would cause muddle if the consultant decided by himself whom to see. In such an open arrangement I would invariably assume a consultative approach on each visit, with the decision to see the child clinically being one which could emerge from the consultation. On the other hand, if the purpose of consultation were primarily training or staff development, it should be an exceptional matter for the consultant to get involved in clinical matters.

This boundary may be crossed unwittingly if the consultant, while not actually seeing the child, occasionally moves from consultative work with the staff (i.e. using their perspectives) to taking a case history and making diagnoses by remote control (i.e. using his own perspectives). Again, while this should be avoided, because it is clinical, not consultative work, it would be absurd for a consultant to refrain from pointing out that a child seems to be at risk for a health or other reason, and to ask appropriate questions, if the consultees seem not to recognise the problem.

If the consultant finds himself taking a clinical case-history he is either being the clinician or being the supervisor. Another way of sliding into the supervisory role is by becoming identified with a particular administrative or political decision. Often, useful consultation will result in the consultees seeing that they have such decisions to make, but it is not for the consultant to indicate what he thinks they should be.

For all these reasons it is important to remember the golden rule of consultation, that if in doubt consult with the consultees. The consultant has no reason whatever to adopt the enigmatic, ambiguous or reticent mien which the occasional psychotherapist seems to find so important. Paradox and mystification have no place in consultation, but the classical psychotherapeutic forms sometimes surface in consultative work because people interested in consultation were often interested in psychotherapy first. But it is a quite different exercise, even though people are sitting about talking problems through.

Ending consultation

The experience of seeing something in a fresh light and the professional development that accompanies it can produce turbulence when the consultee goes back to his own place of work. There are many sorts of consultation where this doesn't arise; circumstances where it can include regular attendance at an outside institution for consultation, or participation in a week's or weekend course. The consultee may then find a conflict between how he or she wants to work, or perceives the organisation, and how colleagues are innocently carrying on.

The consultant should help the consultee foresee what positive and negative effects there could be from what is 'taken home' from consultation, and how to deal with them. The consultee is likely to feel innovative, and this can cause pain. Working in new ways in the old organisation in effect makes the consultee a potential consultant; for example he or she may see a consultative response to an issue or problem where once a directive approach would have been automatic. One of the skills learned by the consultee from useful consultation is how to be a consultant.

Consultation and the community

Many of the practitioners of consultation are psychologists, psychiatrists and social workers, whose empire has in recent years grown wider still and wider. Lipowski (1974, 1977) has pointed out the tremendous potential here for the care and welfare professions to intrude still further into the wider community, ever concerned with the 'promotion of someone else's mental health'. Even though the emphasis of many proponents of consultation, as in this book, is to help widen other people's skills and encourage people to manage with less resort to specialists, nevertheless I believe Lipowski's caution deserves attention, indeed vigilance.

There is a potential ethical dilemma if the consultant is not in sympathy with the consultee's work aims. The reader will be able to think of florid examples of conflict between the moral position of consultant and consultee, but then the consultant would probably avoid becoming involved in the first place. The consultant is more likely to get into difficulties if he or she is ambivalent about the aims and methods of the people or organisation using consultation.

Evaluating consultation

At the moment this is a problem. There have been a number of attempts to evaluate consultative work, but often the work done is not very clearly defined or controlled. Some studies are reviewed in Steinberg and Yule (1985). Interesting findings have included those of Caplan *et al.* (1970) that certain components of consultative work were reported by consultees as more helpful than others, e.g. reduction of theme interference and dealing with stereotypes ('unlinking').

A study of consultative collaboration between a child guidance clinic and a school reported a marked improvement in the children's behaviour though not in intellectual performance or attainment, and noted the teaching staff's initial difficulty with a non-directive consultative approach. They also found that during times of stress, or when new staff joined, there was a shift from consultee-centred work to client-centred work (Woodward *et al.*, 1979). Steinberg and Hughes (1987) reported two separate studies of prolonged work, with child care staff, and with college counsellors, and found in both studies a prominent and sustained shift of emphasis away from client-centred work and towards work-centred consultation. This shift seemed to be initiated by the consultees, who continued to manage their difficult clientele without needing to bring their cases to consultation as frequently as they had at first.

What should be expected of consultation? On the face of it, one hypothesis might be a reduction in direct referrals to specialists and specialist centres, with more of the clientele staying with generalists in 'the community'. On the other hand, attention to the central issue of who should do the right thing for whom could lead to more referrals overall, with more problems coming to light. An outcome most in keeping with the principles of consultation would be not more nor less referrals, but the clientele staying with, or going to, the most appropriate source of help.

Problems with the consultee

One of the assumptions of consultation is that the consultee is a reasonably competent professional, working with integrity in a way appropriate for his experience and seniority. It is because of this act of faith in the consultee that the consultant can proceed with consultation, and not have to become a supervisor or psychotherapist.

Thus, as in examples given earlier, the consultee who recognises his own difficulties in work, areas where he should be better trained, aspects of work he should avoid, or a need for counselling or psychotherapy, is acting responsibly and with competence.

What should the consultant do if a consultee seems unable to recognise, accept or act on the emergence of this sort of information? Clearly the first responsibility of the consultant is to persist with alternative strategies to help the consultee see how his work is being impeded. If the problem persists, however, the consultant may have to consider withdrawing from providing consultation, explaining that the conditions aren't right for a consultative approach, or at least not for the moment. The consultant may have to point out that, for example, supervision, training or a support group may more appropriately meet the individual's or the organisation's needs.

Confidentiality and privacy

Confidentiality and privacy can be harder to maintain for an organisation and its consultees than for patients. A clinician can conceal the identity of a patient in a lecture or published paper without much difficulty. The anonymity of, say, a hospital, a clinic, a school or a social services department is a more difficult matter, because the fact that the consultant operates near 'a teaching hospital' or 'a college of further education' or whatever will certainly lead to inspired guesswork. Of course, it may not matter, and consultees and consultants will often be happy to give each other permission to publish, or present work jointly. Nevertheless, in consultation, issues arise about the effectiveness and efficiency of people and places, and the results of honest self-appraisal could be misrepresented and held against the people concerned.

Occasionally consultants are uneasy when they take their work to a supervisor; should the consultees know that what they say, for example, about colleagues and their organisation is being taken elsewhere? I think they should know, with the reminder that the supervision is about the consultant's work, not about that of the consultees, and that the supervisor must be expected to treat all he or she hears, and of course any notes kept, with complete confidentiality.

The recording of work done, particularly in hospitals, is a current concern, Health Authorities tending to be more impressed by numbers of patients in beds and seen in clinics rather than by those helped 'in the community' by consultative means. Records of consultative work need to be kept as evidence of work done and for other reasons; should they be named according to the professional workers seen or with the name of the client, who after all might be very put out if his name was identifying (or even in) a file in an institution he doesn't attend? My own view is that the file should be kept according to the professional or organisation concerned – with, of course, their knowledge and permission. Client's names should *not* appear.

Finally, changes in the way an organisation operates may seem very exciting and worthwhile to the consultees and their managers; a behavioural programme, for example, may bring about impressive changes in disturbed pupils' behaviour, or a shift from old-fashioned care to a therapeutic milieu, or the introduction of family therapy, may seem like a progressive step for a children's home. I would advise great care with such moves, and either through the managers, or through the consultees, ensure that the privacy of the consultative work is not enabling decisions to by-pass people to whom professional workers should be accountable, not least their clientele.

Chapter 8

Consultation, Creativity and Holistic Medicine

It may seem anomalous to include a chapter about work with patients in a book specifically about work between professionals. In fact both holistic health care and the consultative approach as described here share some basic ethical and practical principles. The holistic approach to medicine will be briefly described before discussing what it has in common with consultation.

Holistic medicine

Holistic medicine means whole person medical and health care. It takes into account the physical, mental and spiritual aspects of the individual and of the total environment. The latter includes the culture as well as physical ecology and family and social relationships, and among the social relationships that influence the diagnosis and management of disorder is the relationship with the doctor or other therapist.

Holistic medicine and health care, undoubtedly fashionable at the moment, also represents some of the better features of traditional medicine, or at least medicine as it has been idealised at its best: the doctor as guide, philosopher, friend and teacher rather than as high-technology specialist alone; though not in the tradition of the doctor as paternalistic authority. Holistic medicine does not dismiss 'alternative' or 'complementary' approaches to healing, nor those which pay attention to the psyche, but neither does it preclude the technical advances medicine and the sciences that contribute to medicine have made.

In this chapter some fundamental principles of holistic medicine are mentioned, and it is suggested that to adopt them requires a creative, imaginative, innovatory approach on the part of both clinician and patient; further, that the consultative approach between professional workers described in this book provides a model for doctor-patient relationships too, and indeed for the work of other therapists as well.

Consider the following clinical vignette. A woman has breast cancer and her family doctor decides to refer her to one of two hospital specialists he knows. One is likely to favour mastectomy, the other would take a more conservative approach, removing only the lump. The general practitioner considers the first surgeon to be the appropriate specialist in the circumstances. The patient would prefer to have the minimum surgical treatment and to see a spiritual healer. The doctor shows, courteously enough, that she doesn't think much of this suggestion, and writes the referral letter.

What are the possible facts of this woman's case, and who is the expert? There is the lump, and who knows what it might do; there is the woman; and there is her family. There is the doctor and the two specialists. They, too, have their individual views, and have interpreted the reports of many years of research from different centres worldwide in rather different ways. They have rarely had the opportunity to examine basic data and the statistics closely, but themselves are influenced by international experts who themselves have differing views.

Then there is the spiritual healer. He may be a crank or a charlatan; or he may be a kindly and supportive person of integrity, working with an aspect of life and faith that could be of real help to the woman; or he could be someone intuitively in touch with an aspect of psychology, physical health and neuro-immunology which clinical science has yet to explore fully (see, for example, Orstein and Sobel, 1988).

Finally, to return to the woman: is she someone expressing her informed and balanced feelings? Or is she so fearful and distressed that she is taking an unjustifiably fatalistic view? What does she understand by spiritual healing? And how much do her family's feelings and opinions matter too?

This example is not particularly complex as medical decisions go. The technical, social, ethical, medico-legal and political issues raised by, for example, AIDS, euthanasia, smoking, drinking alcohol, drug misuse, genetic engineering, artificial insemination, abortion, the detection of disorder *in utero*, organ and tissue transplantation, compulsory treatment for the mentally ill, radiation, food additives, atmospheric lead, toxins in the soil, power cables overhead, the influence of television sex and violence, and the use of drugs that can help and can kill can all generate even more wide-ranging debates, yet decisions have to be reached every day in the consulting room about such matters.

To return to some basic themes of holistic medical practice:

(1) Both the findings of scientific medicine and 'alternative' or 'complementary' approaches are admissible. If something has the reputation of helping some people, from Lourdes to acupuncture or major surgery or tranquillisers it should not be dismissed out of hand.

(2) Not only the patient's mind and body, but the whole person in her total circumstances should be taken into account; not only in terms of diagnosis and treatment, but in how and by whom decisions are made.

(3) The doctor uses intuition and empathy as well as what are traditionally considered the more objective observations. Signs, symptoms and feelings are taken into account, and these include the doctor's feelings and those that arise between doctor and patient.

(4) The doctor starts from where the patient is, beginning as far as possible with *the patient's* language, concepts and wishes.

Given this scope – the whole of life – the doctor and the patient need to be selective and sensible. Real decisions have to be made, but not at the expense of by-passing significant facts, feelings and points of view. The doctor-patient partnership will have to be one that can cope with a new era of attitudes, legislation and technical possibilities, and the complex questions and choices that will accompany it.

Two types of consultation

The first drawing indicates one sort of doctor-patient relationship: the patient is a generator and purveyor of symptoms and

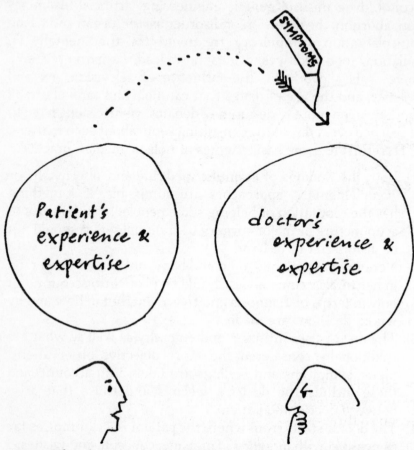

signs. The doctor recognises them, puts them together into a diagnosis or syndrome, and prescribes treatment. Lest this seems to be a hackneyed caricature and repudiation of the traditional medical approach, I have already expressed the view that there are 'holistic' or 'humanistic' practitioners who are critical and dismissive of the 'medical model' yet in fact take this approach themselves, purporting to observe something in the patient they (but not the patient) understand, and offering remedies which, they say, only they can undertake. Lots of progressive and humane people, surgeons and art therapists, physicians and psychotherapists, gynaecologists and marital therapists, psychiatrists and osteopaths, family doctors and family therapists take this approach. Indeed, psychotherapists and counsellors can be every bit as rigid and dogmatic about their theories and methods as the most autocratic of doctors were in days that are fortunately receding.

The second drawing indicates a consultative approach. The

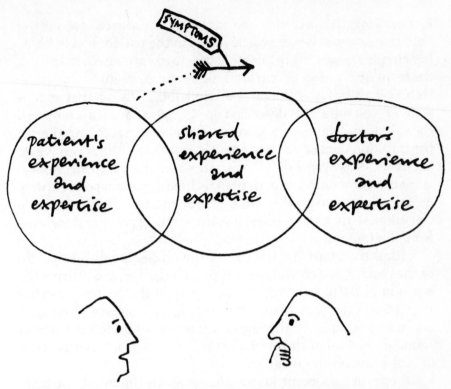

special skills and responsibilities of the doctor (or other specialist) are not abnegated. Instead the doctor, and ideally the patient too, recognise three areas of authority and responsibility:

(1) the clinician as an expert and authority in his or her own speciality, personal views and ethical perspectives;
(2) the patient as an expert and authority on himself or herself, with his or her own ethical and personal preferences;
(3) the responsibility of the doctor to teach and to learn; to help widen the patient's understanding of health, disorder and treatment as the doctor sees it, and in doing so learn more about the patient and the patient's understanding of these things.

There is therefore an exchange of ideas and perspectives in a relationship which helps each help the other to fulfil their respective roles effectively. The patient's responsibility to play his part effectively is no less than the doctor's responsibility to play his.

The task, consistent with the consultative work described throughout this book, is for doctor and patient to pay attention to clarifying the problem and mobilising resources for coping with it; resources which will be found in the patient and in his or her circumstances, from personal beliefs to varieties of help from those in the patient's circle. This is supplemented by those technical things the doctor can contribute, using that extension of consultation described in Chapter 3 as a combined consultative-diagnostic approach. To repeat a recurring theme, the question applied to the patient's problem is 'What can we do about it? What can I do? What can you do? And (if necessary) what can someone else, perhaps a technical specialist or a relative or friend, do?' But this isn't to be intoned as if it were a consultative mantra. Rather, it is the starting point and formula for a joint enquiry.

Rather than blurring the role of the professional and the role of the patient, the consultative approach clarifies and affirms the position of both. Further, the authority of the doctor (or other therapist), far from being diminished, is I believe enhanced, becoming established through mutual consultation on a firmer foundation than authority by tradition, by accident, or because of a diploma on the wall.

Of course the doctor knows things about the mind, the body and medicines that the patient may not, and this information is for sharing. But the patient knows things about himself and his situation that the doctor cannot know; he is indeed the expert on himself. Just as important, they can put their heads together about those areas of medicine and the person that aren't known. The doctor acts as teacher, which is an archetypal function of the doctor as well as the meaning of the word.

The better teachers learn new things all the time, not least from their students, and often use a consultative style, helping the student find out for himself. The point has often been made in many different contexts that the phenomenal expansion of information in all fields means that now the most important thing for teachers to teach is how to learn. The technical, cultural and ethical matters, dilemmas and conundra with which questions of health and medicine are riddled means that the most productive way forward is as a joint patient-doctor concern. (Concern is itself an interesting word, meaning sifting together.)

The holistic approach: concluding note

'Holistic' refers to the whole person in context. Consultation provides a way in to this approach to health care in a way that is essentially simple and straightforward, and proceeds step by step, yet allows for all the personal, social, cultural, medico-technical, medico-legal and ethical questions that could arise. But it is not over-inclusive; at each step priorities and realities are sorted out, and common sense (i.e that understanding which is common to those involved), and jointly agreed expediency, can

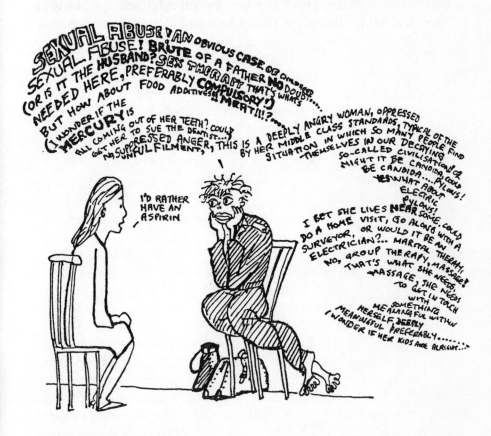

certainly take precedence over what each participant believes (or even fears) is as it were ideologically or technically 'correct'. In this sense consultation is genuinely liberating, unlike some currently fashionable ideologies which operate like mental straitjackets and can conflict with what individuals believe in their hearts is right.

For reasons already argued, consultation does not diminish the authority of the expert, but on the contrary puts it into a sounder relationship with the natural authority of the patient. In this respect the relationship proposed here between physician and patient is similar to that which has developed in recent years in *some* approaches to counselling, psychotherapy, and family therapy as well as in holistic medical practice.

The point is not to blur the boundaries but to shift them, in a way which pays attention to the expertise of the supposedly less expert. It is because this is the territory of interprofessional consultation that it also has a bearing on relationships between professional workers and their clientele.

Chapter 9

Working Together: Consultation, Collaboration and Creativity

The means to act

The point of consultation is effective action, whether in dealing with a clinical crisis or planning a course of training. This is achieved by seeking to place in the right positions the appropriate authority, the proper responsibility, the relevant information and skills, and sufficient confidence and motivation.

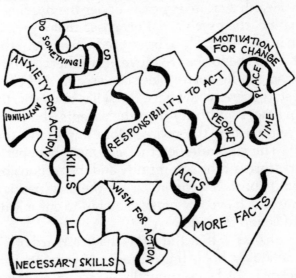

It is because these things are often all over the place that difficulties arise, and that consultation is useful.

Example: A social worker provides the following information. A seventeen-year-old girl is leading a grossly self-negligent life, in and out of her parents' home, on which she still depends, but spending long periods in squats where she is exploited. She has taken several overdoses, dabbled in drug abuse, been arrested for drunkenness and is putting herself at risk from AIDS.

The parents feel responsibility but have insufficient effective authority. The Social Services Department have considered taking care proceedings, but are reluctant to take this action with a seventeen-year-old, and lack the skills and resources to help her if she were in care. Attempts at counselling, including the use of informal self-help groups, and family therapy, were ineffectual because of the girl's reluctance to use them.

There are no police charges outstanding and she is currently breaking no laws, so there is no way of enforcing any preventive or remedial action through the Courts.

One of the questions that brings her case to consultation is whether admission to a psychiatric hospital will help. However, she refuses even to consider this, and it is concluded that there are no grounds to enforce admission by using the Mental Health Act. In any case, under the heading 'skills and information' the psychiatrist proposes that a period of treatment in hospital is likely to be unproductive; if anything would help, it would be for her to move into a therapeutic community – a home or hostel for older adolescents and young adults.

The staff there would have the skills; however, they do not have any more authority than the parents, the social worker, the psychiatrist or the police. More important, they do not want it. The communities that are available operate by the peer-pressures of the community and the responsibility to the community of each resident. Use of the therapeutic communities may be achieved by persuasion but to enforce it would be a contradiction in terms.

The outcome is that the girl is made a Ward of Court. The Court, uniquely, holds the authority to insist that she accepts help, despite not being mentally ill, accepting the argument that although her liberty is being interfered with against her wishes, her immaturity justifies a last chance of asserting adult pressure in a way that could save her life and health. There will not be another opportunity for such paternalism, and in a year or two she can be free to take these risks herself.

The case, which through her own solicitor the client doesn't argue against with any vigour, hinges on her immaturity and being at risk.

With the authority of the Court, the moral responsibility of the parents and the executive responsibility of the Social Services Department, the girl is required to stay for a time in hospital to see whether the therapeutic environment and the presence of other young people might help persuade her that a therapeutic hostel would after all be worth trying.

This does not succeed, and in due course the girl returns to her old way of life, after which things get worse.

There can be many permutations of these ingredients – authority, responsibility, information and motivation. At one extreme, for example an acutely psychotic patient treated compulsorily as an emergency in hospital, all may rest for a time in the psychiatrist, and in due course be shared with the nearest relatives.

At the other extreme, to refer again to the points made when consultation was compared with Rogerian counselling, and with holistic medicine, the therapist acts as teacher; authority, responsibility, information, motivation and the confidence to act then all become part of the repertoire of the patient. (Or erstwhile patient; because when this shift has taken place effectively he or she can discard that role.)

Between these extremes there are many occasions in day to day work when consultation demonstrates relatively simple ways by which the work several people are doing can be done more effectively by clarifying roles and responsibilities.

Example: To take a straightforward example, a teenage boy with a long history of deprivation, unhappiness and misbehaviour, and frequent changes in those looking after him, now has a psychiatrist, a social worker, and two or three care staff in his children's home seeing him irregularly and informally for support, advice, counselling and limit-setting. The work isn't going well and all concerned feel deskilled, and wish he could see a psychotherapist; but there isn't one available. It appears very much as if the staff are responding to the adolescent's low self-esteem and pessimism by tending to go along with his belief that no adult will ever be good enough to help him.

The following proposals come out of a consultative session: that one of the care staff takes on a regular, more systematic counselling role focussed on his feelings and relationships, and this work is supervised by the psychiatrist. The psychiatrist limits her own direct contact with the teenager to occasional assessments of his progress. The social worker changes the focus of his work from *ad hoc* counselling and support to asserting the authority *in loco parentis* invested in the Care Order, making clear his backing for the efforts of the children's home staff and the psychiatrist.

The other care staff concentrate more on making sure that the boy participates properly in the life of the home. They remain open and friendly towards him, but now direct his request for talking sessions, previously indiscriminately sought, lengthy, unproductive and apparently unsatisfying to the boy himself, to the twice-weekly sessions with his counsellor.

The boy finds himself no longer in control of a number of uncertain-seeming adults, but instead finds confident, competent people in charge of him. After a brief flurry of half-hearted protest at the new arrangements, things begin to improve.

What had gone somewhat awry is common, though in very variable degrees, throughout the whole field of psychiatric, psychological and social work. Relatively little is known for certain about the best ways of working, and indeed the nature of many of the questions involved is such that there cannot be any clear-cut or uncontroversial answer. People tend to bring to their work quite different sources of authority on what to do for their clientele: this may be the institute they trained in, a teacher or writer who has impressed them, their own senior, or it may be based on a personal belief and value system. To this inflammable mixture may be added the igniting effect of the pressure for quick, sure and correct solutions to extremely difficult human problems. The core difficulty is that so complex are the problems in these fields that different perspectives and skills are essential, and yet they may sit uneasily alongside each other, challenging organisation, leadership and decision-making (see Steinberg, 1986a).

The result may be a creative, productive tension, or

destructive conflict. Quite commonly there is neither, and instead a quiet collusion in chronic mild underfunctioning and disorganisation at best, or disillusionment, pessimism and helplessness at worst. As I have emphasised elsewhere (Steinberg, 1981) this is not because personnel in these fields are inherently incompetent, but because the work is extremely demanding, and in some of the most difficult areas staff are relatively poorly led, trained, supervised, looked after, provided for and paid. Consultation is not a panacea, but can provide a way into sorting this multiplicity of problems one from another, assisting discussion and co-operation, and encouraging joint enquiry into what is possible and sensible. Consultation may be available in any of the ways outlined in Chapter 2 (Figure 2.2), but there is a further important category, when with training, professional development and maturity staff members automatically adopt a consultative style in their dealings with each other, and indeed with experience can in due course consult with themselves.

From babble to Babel

'REPORT DAMNS SEX ABUSE BATTLEGROUND' were the headlines on one of the more sober and restrained British newspapers when the inquiry chaired by Lord Justice Butler-Sloss reported its findings (HMSO, 1988a). In a small area of England and over a short period of time one hundred and twenty-one children were taken into care, suspected of being sexually abused, often as emergency action and apparently with much emphasis on two doctors' interpretation of a physical sign, reflex anal dilatation, about which the Standing Medical Advisory Committee for the Department of Health and Social Security commented: 'It cannot be emphasised too strongly that no physical sign can at the present time be regarded as uniquely diagnostic of child sexual abuse' (HMSO, 1988b).

The cases and subsequent report generated a great deal of media comment, some better informed than others, and it is difficult to know what precisely went on during this extraordinary episode. It did seem that the doctors were acting according to one set of assumptions about the clinical evidence for sexual abuse, that their concern and efforts were matched by the

Department of Social Services' child sex abuse expert, who was reported as being sceptical about the value of working with families.

In the report strong differences of view between agencies (the various doctors, the police and the social services) were noted, as was the absence of efforts to bring them together; words such as 'rifts' and 'deadlock' were used to describe relationships between the police and the social services; the legal division of the local authority seemed little consulted, even on such matters as parents' access to their children or their right to second medical opinions; controversy over the validity of such medical information and knowledge as existed was acknowledged in the Report, but did not appear to have made much impact during the months when children were being rushed into care on Place of Safety Orders. Parents appeared isolated from what was going on, as were other professionals and agencies who might have been able to help, or who had other opinions. In consultative terms, responsibility, authority and the necessary information and skills seemed to have a skewed distribution. The Report called for, among other things, better inter-agency training and cooperation.

From time to time such inter-professional crises emerge, usually over a dramatic issue such as children being taken into care *en masse* or conversely not being protected at all, or when a Department of Social Services falls apart or a doctor is suspended. In fact, lesser degrees of failed collaboration are very common, particularly where problems are complex and multifaceted (e.g. with ethical as well as clinical components), where the facts are scanty or open to different interpretations, and where several people, professions or agencies need to work together. All this applies very much to the type of work discussed throughout this book.

Why should tension and conflict arise so readily in these fields? It is partly a matter of the differences of opinion already mentioned, and endemic and inevitable in this work. Dispute can no more be avoided here than it could be in, say, a healthy legal or political system. The difference, however, is that instead of these complex questions being debated in the relative calm and security of a Court of Law or Parliamentary Debating Chamber, or in the luxury and freedom of a journalist's column, they have to be sorted out swiftly by the person or people on the spot in a busy clinic or office, with other people waiting and the telephone ringing, and sometimes on the doorstep.

For one reasonably experienced person to act by himself or herself may be merely difficult. But when the situation demands more than one sort of expertise (for example, psychiatrist, paediatrician, social worker and police officer) the difficulties can become horrendous and near impossible. Each will have developed his or her own way, emotionally and professionally, of managing challenging situations; many of these strategies will have been formalised in the operational guidelines and instructions of their own organisations, professions, indeed in their basic training. To cope with the other professionals on top of coping with the core crisis may be the last straw, and result in mutual anger and chaos. In practice, people have the foresight to see this coming, so that while the occasional chaotic breakdown of services may hit the headlines, what is far more common in practice is collusion in avoidance; avoidance of a particular type of client, or issue, or practitioner. So the behavioural scientists organise their working lives so as not to bandy words with psychoanalysts, certain sorts of psychologists and psychiatrists keep out of each other's way in the interests of self-management of tension and blood pressure, social workers and police officers politely skirt about important questions in order to keep the peace. These things go on, to the detriment of services, training and the clientele. Indeed, it is because good routine collaboration between people with different expertise and approaches is the exception rather than the rule, that when things do go visibly wrong they tend to do so on a grand scale.

We hold on tight to what we know, in a way that has echoes of the attachment model discussed earlier. Mature, thinking, reflective Man is as uncomfortable on the boundaries of his personal knowledge and assumptions as was the toddler venturing near the boundary of the territory that parent and child together feel is safe. The acceptance of new ideas, which includes, of course, other people's old ideas, is treated with the same hesitation that protected us a long time ago, and still does, from chewing naively on poisonous plants. This caution has a strong and useful pedigree; we don't swallow new things too readily.

The exploration of new ideas and the acquisition of new information has its tensions and its territory. Scientists and philosophers advance with the exquisite care of mountaineers, as anxious about the integrity of their methodology as are serious climbers about their equipment. The speculative, intuitive thinkers who bound along without visible means of support are seen as the Bugs Bunnies of the field, causing irritation and envy when they receive (undeserved) recognition, and some satisfaction when they jump over the edge. On the other hand, they may get a better view. The point is that these feelings and their pre-rational origins are no less powerfully influential in the most conscientious of scientists than in the most imaginative speculators, and they get in the way, one way or another, of effective collaboration. Everybody knows he or she is right.

Consultation, innovation and creativity

Consultation is joint exploration. As to what is explored, this has been the substance of much of the preceding pages. It is partly a matter of exploring the question at hand, partly exploring the alternatives for managing it, and partly exploring what there is in oneself, in the consultative relationship and in the work setting that helps the work advance.

The joint nature of the exercise implies, in consultation, more than simply working together. The consultant's respect for the consultee's perspective should be genuine; indeed, he or she will depend on it, and be curious about it. In helping with the consultee's work, the consultant should find in the consultee a valuable instrument, on a par with the radio telescope or electron microsope or the latest imaging devices, for seeing something in a new way and making new discoveries. But the consultant helps the consultee use his or her instrumental capacities. It should be a truly joint enterprise, and the more real the differences in perspective the better the view – that is, if this binocular instrument is used properly.

A recurring theme in the literature of creativity is the innovatory power of bringing together different, opposite or contradictory ideas or images (e.g. Arieti, 1976). Rothenberg has referred to this as Janusian thinking (Rothenberg, 1971) from Janus, a Roman deity with origins in Greece, who was custodian of the universe and looked inward and outward from its gate, symbolic of duality and of the wholeness in opposites. He developed into the god of beginnings; hence January. The theme persists in mythology and literature, in dialectical logic and reasoning in which contradictory ideas lead to further developments in thinking. We may perceive its biological roots in that crucial stage of evolution represented by meiosis, through which sexual reproduction (as opposed to the asexual reproduction of primitive forms of life) allows new individuals of infinite variety to develop. At a social level, and returning again to collaborative efforts, studies have been made of the relationship between the creative efforts of individuals and their work in pairs and groups (Triandis, 1963; Triandis *et al.* 1965). The implications are complex but the principle simple: once you move from one perspective, dimension or form to two or more, the potential for innovation becomes enormous, providing the alternatives come together constructively. Consultation proceeds as if in a double spiral, one strand attentive, intellectual and enquiring, the other to do with a relationship which combines curiosity, tension and confidence in a creative, constructive state not far removed from play. Each turn of the cycle of questions and answers leads to higher ground, at which level more finely tuned questions and answers can be formulated.

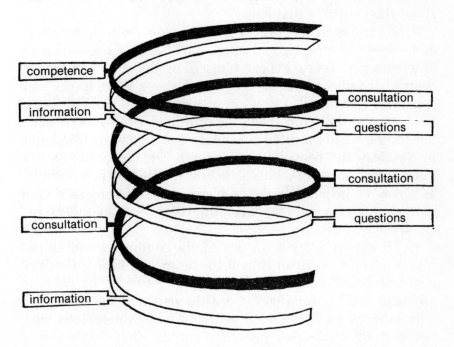

Consultation and the future

The present age is one of specialisation and highly technical education, but people's knowledge of what each other do, even the work of the person next door or in the next room, often appears limited. High levels of education and sophistication (and there's a word with interesting origins) do not guarantee a sound grasp of how the world works, whether biologically, socially, economically or psychologically. From a more parochial perspective, and back to the theme of this book, the researcher who sought to study how far professionals working in the same area or even in the same organisation or department had a good enough grasp of each other's perspective would have some surprises, and some interesting findings.

But people's needs and problems aren't specialised. They come in complex, vague and sometimes messy amalgams of physical, economic, domestic, psychological, cultural and social factors, often involving difficult questions to do with dependence and independence of choice and action. This in turn requires encouraging as much self-help as possible, and where specialised help is necessary, that people are as fully educated as possible about the nature of that help.

If the various professions, of which there are many, are to help each other and other people with what little they know (and it's little enough) every expert himself or herself needs to be somewhat Janus-faced, looking to whatever their special skill happens to be but also to ways of recognising, mobilising and inspiring the skills and strengths of others. Both sets of skills, one technical and the other consultative, should go hand in hand. In this way the consultative approach can not only enhance interprofessional work, but can operate in the wider community as a way of helping clarify problems and solutions as a joint enterprise, and in ways that everyone concerned can understand and use.

As far as psychiatry is concerned, the continuing widespread review of how best to respond to the mental health needs of populations and communities is amply justified. The types of problems and treatments, the practitioners and the settings in which they work represent an extraordinarily variegated range; nor is it either clear or generally agreed which problems of human life, development and behaviour are or are not 'psychiatric'. While a degree of nebulousness is to be expected, there is also a lot of wasteful muddle. There does seem to be general agreement that the question of who does what for whom, and with what skills and facilities, needs thorough re-examination.

One way of doing this is through philosophy and semantics, another is by distributing acres of questionnaires. Another, very popular at present, is by drawing up grand designs on paper for complex networks of relationships between offices, agencies and personnel and giving the latter new titles.

Instead of these, I would like to suggest that the wider use and teaching of the consultative approach, designed as it is to educate the consultant in what is wanted, the consultee in what is needed, and both in what is possible, all at a personal, local and pragmatic level, would help clear up some of the chaos and point out some useful directions with a pertinence, precision and economy that large scale planning cannot achieve.

References and Bibliography

Arieti, S. (1976). *Creativity*. New York: Basic Books.

Balint, M. (1968) *The Doctor, His Patient and the Illness*. London: Pitman.

Bennet, G. (1979) *Patients and Their Doctors*. London: Baillière Tindall.

Bennet, G. (1987) *The Wound and the Doctor*. London: Secker and Warburg.

Bergan, J.R. and Tombari, M.L. (1976) Consultant skill and efficiency and the implementation and outcomes of consultation. *Journal of School Psychology* **14**, 3–41.

Berger, M. (1979) Behaviour modification in education and professional practice: the danger of mindless technology. *Bulletin of the British Psychological Society*, **32**, 418–419.

Berlin, I. (1969) Mental health consultation for school social workers: a conceptual model. *Community Mental Health Journal*, **5, 4**, 280–288.

Berlin, I.N. (1965) Mental health consultation in the schools: who can do it and why. *Community Health Journal* **1**, 19–22.

Bindmann, A.J. (1966) The clinical psychologist as a mental health consultant. In *Progress in Clinical Psychology*. New York: Grune & Stratton.

Brown, D. and Pedder, J. (1979) *Introduction to Psychotherapy*. London: Tavistock.

Bowlby, J. (1969) *Attachment and Loss. Volume 1: Attachment*. London: Hogarth Press.

Bowlby, J. (1973) *Attachment and Loss. Volume 2: Separation:* Anxiety and Anger. London: Hogarth Press.

Bowlby, J. (1980) *Attachment and Loss. Volume 3: Loss*. London: Hogarth Press.

Bruggen, P., Byng-Hall, J. and Pitt-Aikens, T. (1973) The reason for admission as a focus of work for an adolescent unit. *British Journal of Psychiatry* **122**, 319–329.

Caplan, G. (1964) *Principles of Preventive Psychiatry*. London: Tavistock.

Caplan, G. (1970) *The Theory and Practice of Mental Health Consultation*. London: Tavistock.

Caplan, G., Howe, L.P. and Owens, C. (1970) Study reported in Caplan, G. (1970) *The Theory and Practice of Mental Health Consultation*, pp. 301–327. London: Tavistock.

Conoley, J.C. (ed.) (1981) *Consultation in Schools: Theory, Research, Procedures*. New York: Academic Press.

Conoley, J.C. (1981) Emergent training issues in consultation. In Conoley, J.C. (ed.) *Consultation in Schools: Theory, Research, Procedures*. New York: Academic Press.

Conoley, J.C. and Conoley, C.W. (1982). *School Consultation: A Guide to Practice and Training*. New York: Pergamon.

Dare, C. (1986) Family therapy and an in-patient unit. In Steinberg, D. (ed.) *The Adolescent Unit: Work and Teamwork in Adolescent Psychiatry*. pp. 83–95. Chichester: John Wiley.

Dare, C. (1982) Techniques of Consultation. In Dare, C., Ryle, R., Steinberg, D. and Yule, W. (eds.) Consultation from Child and Adolescent Psychiatric Clinics and an ILEA Child Guidance Unit. *News of the Association of Child Psychology and Psychiatry*, **11**, 1–16.

Dare, C. (1983) Clinical Work with Children in Care. Paper presented at the Royal College of Psychiatrists' Child and Adolescent Psychiatry Section, Spring Scientific Meeting. Unpublished.

Dare, C., Ryle, R., Steinberg, D and Yule, W. (1982) Training for consultation. In Dare, C., Ryle, R., Steinberg, D. and Yule, W. (eds.) Consultation from Child and Adolescent Psychiatric Clinics and an ILEA Child Guidance Unit. *News of the Association of Child Psychology and Psychiatry*, **11**, 1–16.

Dorr, D. (1979) Psychological consulting in the schools. In Platt, J.J. and Wicks, R.J. (eds.) *The Psychological Consultant*. New York: Grune and Stratton.

Etzioni, A. (1968) *Modern Organisations*, New York: Prentice Hall.

Foskett, J. (1986) The Staff Group. In Steinberg, D. (ed.) *The Adolescent Unit. Work and Teamwork in Adolescent Psychiatry*. pp. 169–178 Chichester: John Wiley.

French, W.L. and Bell, C.H. (1973) *Organisation Development*. New Jersey: Prentice Hall.

Gallessich, J. (1974) Training the school psychologist for consultation. *Journal of School Psychology*, **12, 2**, 138–149.

Gallessich, J. (1982) *The Profession and Practice of Consultation: a handbook for consultants, trainers of consultants and consumers of consultation services*. London: Jossey-Bass.

Gelder, M., Gath, D. and Mayou, R. (1985). *Oxford Textbook of Psychiatry*. Oxford: Oxford University Press.

Georgiades, N.J. and Phillimore, L. (1975) The myth of the hero-innovator and alternative strategies for organisational change. In Kiernan, C.C. and Woodford, F. (eds.) *Behaviour Modification with the Severely Retarded*. Amsterdam: Associated Scientific Publishers.

Gomez, J. (1986) *Liaison Psychiatry*. London: Croom Helm.

Harvey, L., Kolvin, I., McLaren, M., Nicol, A.R. and Wolstenholme, F. (1977). Introducing a school social worker into schools. *British Journal of Guidance and Counselling*, **5 (1)**, 26–40.

Heard, D.H. (1974) Crisis intervention guided by attachment concepts – a case study. *Journal of Child Psychology and Psychiatry*, **15**, 111–22.

Heard, D.H. (1978) From object relations to attachment theory: a basis for family therapy. *British Journal of Medical Psychology*, **51**, 67–76.

Her Majesty's Stationery Office (1988a) *The Report of the Inquiry into Child Abuse in Cleveland*. London: HMSO.

Her Majesty's Stationery Office (1988b) *Diagnosis of Child Sexual Abuse: guidance for doctors*. London: HMSO.

Jason, L.A., Ferone, L. and Anderegg, T. (1979) Evaluating ecological, behavioural and process consultation interventions. *Journal of School Psychology*, **17 (2)**, 103–115.

Jennings, S. (1981) *Remedial Drama*. London: A. and C. Black.

Jennings, S. (1985) (ed.) *Creative Therapy*. Banbury, Oxon: Kemble Press.

Jennings, S. (1986) *Creative Drama in Group Work*. London: Winslow Press.

Jones, M. (1970) Social learning in methods of teaching psychiatry. In Russell, G.F.M. and Walton, H.J. (eds.). The Training of Psychiatrists. *British Journal of Psychiatry Special Publication, No 5*. pp. 64–65. Ashford, Kent: Headley Brothers Ltd.

Keys, C.B. Organisation development: An Approach to Mental Health Consultation. In Mannino, F.V., Trickett, E.J., Shore, M.F., Kedder, M.G. and Levin G. (eds.) (1986) Handbook of Mental Health Consultation. Washington D.C: U.S. Department of Health and Human Services.

Kolvin, I., Garside, R.F., Nicol, A.R., MacMillan, A., Wolstenholme, F. and Leitch, I.M. (1981) *Help Starts Here: The Malajusted Child in the Ordinary School*. London: Tavistock.

Lambert, N.M., Yandell, W. and Sandoval, J.H. (1975) Preparation of school psychologists for school-based consultation: a training activity and a service to community schools. *Journal of School Psychology*, **13 (1)**, 63–75.

Lewin, K. (1952) *Field Theory in Social Science*. London: Tavistock.

Likert, R. (1961) *New Patterns of Management*. New York: McGraw.

Lipowski, Z.J. (1974) Consultation-liaison psychiatry: an overview. *American Journal of Psychiatry*, **131 (6)**, 623–630.

Lipowski, Z.J. (1977) Psychiatric consultation: concepts and controversies. *American Journal of Psychiatry*, **134 (5)**, 523–528.

Lyons, S. and Tropea, E. (1987) Creative arts therapists as consultants: methods and approaches to inservice training in the special education forum. *The Arts In Psychotherapy*, **14**, 243–247.

Mannino, F. and Shore, M. (1975) The effects of consultation: a review of empirical studies. *American Journal of Community Psychology*, **3**, 1–21.

Martin, R. and Myers, J. (1980) School psychologists and the practice of Consultation *Psychology in Schools*, **17**, 478–484.

Menzies, I. (1970) The functioning of social systems as a defence against anxiety. London: Tavistock Institute of Human Relations, Pamphlet No 3.

Menzies, I. (1974) Staff support systems. Task and Antitask in adolescent institutions. *Proceedings of the Ninth Annual Conference of the Association for the Psychiatric Study of Adolescence*, 13–22.

Meyers, J. (1981) Mental Health Consultation. In Conoley, J.C. (ed.) *Consultation in Schools: Theory, Research, Procedures*. New York: Academic Press.

Meyers, J. Parson, R.D. and Martin, R. (1979) *Mental Health Consultations in the School*. San Francisco: Jossey Bass.

Meyers, J., Wurtz, R. and Flanagan, D. (1981) A national survey investigating consultation training occuring in school psychology programs. *Psychology in Schools*, **18**, 297–302.

Meyers, J., Pitt, N., Gaughan, E. and Friedman, M. (1978) A research model for consultation with teachers. *Journal of School Psychology*, **16**, 137–145.

Mrazek, D. (1985) Child psychiatric consultation and liaison to paediatrics. In Rutter, M. and Hersov, L. *Child & Adolescent Psychiatry: Modern Approaches*, 888–899. Oxford: Blackwell Scientific Publications.

Orstein, R. and Sobel, D. (1988) *The Healing Brain*. London: MacMillan.

Palazzoli, M.S. (1984) Behind the scenes of the organisation: some guidelines for the expert in human relations. *Journal of Family Therapy*, **6**, 299–307.

Pipes, R.B. (1981) Consulting the organisations: the entry problem. In Conoley, J.C. (ed.) *Consultation in Schools: Theory, Research, Procedures*. London: Academic Press.

Plog, S.C. (1977) Effectiveness, leadership and consultation. In Plog S.C. and Ahmed, P.H. (eds.) *Principles and Techniques of Mental Health Consultation*. New York: Plenum Press.

Reder, P. and Kraemer, S. (1980) Dynamic aspects of professional collaboration in child guidance referral. *Journal of Adolescence*, **3**, 165–173.

Ritter, D.R. (1978) Effects of a school consultation program upon referral patterns of teachers. *Psychology in Schools*, **15**, 239–243.

Rogers, C. (1951) *Client-centered Therapy*. Boston, Massachusetts: Houghton-Mifflin Company.

Rothenberg, A. (1971) The process of Janusian thinking in creativity. *Archives of General Psychiatry*, **24**, 185–205.

Ryle, R. (1982) Understanding organisations. In Dare, C., Ryle, R., Steinberg, D. and Yule, W. (eds). *News of the Association of Child Psychology and Psychiatry*, **11**, 1–16.

Sandler, J. (1976) Counter-transference and role-responsiveness. *International Review of Psychoanalysis*, **3**, 43–47.

Sandler, J., Dare, C. and Holder, A. (1970). Basic psychoanalytic concepts: III. Transference. *British Journal of Psychiatry*, **116**, 667–672.

Skynner, A.C.R. (1964) Group-analytic themes in training and case discussion groups. In *Selected Lectures: Sixth International Congress of Psychotherapy*. Basle: Karger.

Skynner, A.C.R. (1974) An experiment in group consultation with the staff of a comprehensive school. *Group Process*, **6**, 99–114.

Skynner, A.C.R. (1975) The large group in training. In Kreeger, L. (ed) *The Large Group*. London: Constable 227–251.

Steinberg, D. (1981) Using Child Psychiatry: the functions and operations of a specialty. London: Hodder & Stoughton.

Steinberg, D. (1982) Treatment, training, care or control? *British Journal of Psychiatry*, **141**, 306–309.

Steinberg, D. (1983) *The Clinical Psychiatry of Adolescence: Clinical work from a social and developmental perspective.* Chichester: John Wiley.

Steinberg, D. (1986a) (ed) *The Adolescent Unit: Work and Teamwork in Adolescent Psychiatry.* Chichester: John Wiley.

Steinberg, D. (1986b) Psychiatric aspects of problem behaviour: a consultative approach. In Tattum, D. (ed.) Management of disruptive pupil behaviour in schools, 187–205. Chichester: John Wiley

Steinberg, D. (1987) *Basic Adolescent Psychiatry.* Oxford: Blackwell Scientific Publications.

Steinberg, D. (1988) Management of crises and emergencies. In Hsu, L. and Herson, M. *Recent Developments in Adolescent Psychiatry.* New York: John Wiley.

Steinberg, D. (1989) The Imagination in therapy: Consultative and creative approaches in holistic care. In Kareem, J. and Littlewood, R. (eds.) Intercultural therapy, theory and techniques. Oxford: Blackwell Scientific Publications: in preparation.

Steinberg, D. and Yule, W. (1985) Consultative work. In Rutter M. and Hersov, L. (eds.) *Child and Adolescent Psychiatry: Modern Approaches.* 914–926. Oxford: Blackwell Scientific Publications.

Steinberg, D. and Hughes, L. (1987) The emergence of work-centred issues in consultative work: an observation. *Journal of Adolescence,* **10**, 309–316.

Tattum, D. (1986a) (ed.) *Management of Disruptive Pupil Behaviour in Schools.* Chichester: John Wiley.

Tattum, D. (1986b) (ed.) Consistency management – school and classroom concerns. In Tattum, D. (1986) (ed.) *Management of Disruptive Pupil Behaviour in Schools.* pp. 51–68. Chichester: John Wiley.

Tharp, R.G. and Wetzel, R.J. (1969) *Behaviour Modification in the Natural Environment.* New York: Academic Press.

Topping, K. (1986) Consultative enhancement of school-based action. In Tattum, D. (1986) (ed.) *Management of Disruptive Pupil Behaviour in Schools.* pp. 31–50. Chichester: John Wiley.

Triandis, H.C. (1963) Team creativity as a function of the creativity of the members. *Journal of Applied Psychology,* **47**, 104–110.

Triandis, H.C., Hall, E.R. and Ewen, R.B. (1965) Member heterogeneity and dyadic creativity. *Human Relations,* **18**, 33–55.

Tyrer, P. and Steinberg, D. (1987) *Models for Mental Disorder: Conceptual Models in Psychiatry.* Chichester: John Wiley.

Wigley, V., Yule, W. and Berger, M. (1982). A primary solution to soiling. *Special Education* **9** (4), 27–30.

Wilson, P. (1986) Individual psychotherapy in a residential setting. In Steinberg, D. (ed.) *The Adolescent Unit: Work and Teamwork in Adolescent Psychiatry.* pp. 97–111. Chichester: John Wiley.

Woodward, C.A., Johnson, J., Santa-Barbara, J., Roberts, R.S. and Pipe, M. (1979) A collaboration special educational program for emotionally disturbed children: philosophy, design and outcomes. In Shamsie, S.J. (ed.) *New Directions in Children's Mental Health.* pp. 41–51. New York: SP Medical & Scientific Books.

Yule, W. (1982) Some examples of consultative work. In Dare, C., Ryle, R.

Steinberg, D. and Yule, W. (eds.) Consultation from Child and Adolescent Psychiatric Settings and an ILEA Child Guidance Unit. *News of the Association of Child Psychology and Psychiatry.* **11**, 1–16.

Yule, W., Berger, M. and Wigley, V. (1977). The teacher-child interaction project. *Bulletin of the British Association of Behaviour Psychotherapists*, **5 (3)**, 42–47.

Yule, W., Berger, M. and Wigley, V. (1983) Behaviour modification and classroom management. In Frude, N. and Gault, H. (eds.) *Children at School.* Chichester: John Wiley.

Index